I0463179

When The Time Comes

Nursing Home Guide

Also by Elaine Stubbs

Dandelions in December

To Follow A Dream

Elaine Stubbs

When The Time Comes

Nursing Home Guide

All rights reserved

ISBN-13: 978-1463573768

ISBN-10: 1463573766

Dedication

I dedicate *When The Time Comes ~ Nursing Home Guide* to you, the reader, in hopes that all your experiences with nursing homes will be positive. It also is dedicated to my daughter, Liana, who has ever encouraged me through three books, to my son Daren and his wife Teri, and my much loved one-and-only grandchild, Katie. It would not be possible to leave one of my lifetime friends off this list. Her name is Theresa Brewer, R.N.

Contents

Author's Note

This book is for all those who may have to enter, or place a loved one in a skilled nursing home. It comes from someone who has twenty-seven years of experience "in the trenches" as a director of nursing, administrator, regional manager and consultant in long-term care facilities, commonly known as nursing homes, reaching across the country. I have witnessed many, many family members' joy, tragedy, discouragement and elation in my nursing homes and I have learned from each of them.

This is also for those who will feel or have felt the aching, pounding guilt because you had no other choice but a nursing home for your loved one. I dealt with the guilt of family members every day of my career. I understood the guilt and I understood the fear and concerns. They were entrusting a person that they loved very dearly to people they didn't know. Besides that, they had heard all the horror stories. Would all of these terrible things befall them and their loved one?

If you are the caretaker of a loved one, there may come a time when you have reached the final limit. This is mostly guaranteed to happen unless the caregiver has devoted their entire life and future to the loved one. This does happen but most people cannot endure the physical and mental stress of the never-ending care and problems that go along with tending to their loved one's needs. It could be your very ill mother, incontinent of both bowel and bladder that requires feeding and total care. How long can you keep up the 24-hour job? You have a spouse and maybe even children that need attention and support from you. You will know when the time comes to do something. You can find no way around putting your loved one in a nursing home. You experience tremendous guilt; you lose sleep. But in the end, it's the only thing than can be done.

The very ill can benefit from nursing home care at a good facility. Of course, there are also residents in nursing facilities who are recovering from surgery, are involved in extensive daily therapy and of course, the Alzheimer's victims and the grossly confused who benefit as well. Other patients with less severe problems can be admitted to assisted living centers until the required nursing care has surpassed the center's skills and licensing. There are bad assisted living centers just like there are bad hospitals and bad nursing homes. **You've got to do your homework.**

Through this writing, I will attempt to acquaint you with how a good nursing home is run, how to tour a nursing home and what to look for. There will be tips and a few stories along the way.

It is my hope that you will realize that the nursing home experience doesn't have to be a horror story, and that you will know you have the ability to find the right place for your loved one.

So, come along with me. It won't be complicated and as I said, I've included some of my stories to make it easier to understand. The last thing I want is for this work to be as dry as a textbook. You will find many facts repeated in this book. I've done this on purpose as there are always many different contexts. My main purpose is to help you find the nursing home right for you and your loved one, break down the fear of nursing homes and relieve some of the guilt trips so very common in family members. Only with a positive attitude can you and your loved one make the nursing home experience a good one. I will always urge you to do your homework in selecting the long-term care facility that is right for you and/or your loved one.

This is for you.

Chapter One

The Purpose of These Words

A man visited my office during the time I was opening a new long-term care center in Ft. Myers, Florida. He was tall and very handsome with sandy hair. I figured him for an architect. He stood in the doorway of my office until I invited him in. This was real "class" as most family members barge right in and plop down on the sofa while talking non-stop. He had just admitted his mother to my new nursing home and said he had some words for me. He came in and sat down. I had no idea what would come next. A serious complaint? But no. He came to tell me I wasn't doing my job. I straightened up at this and peered, owl-eyed, at him across the desk.

He said, "Let me tell you what I mean. Both my wife and I are professionals but we had no foreknowledge of what to expect when we came to admit my mother.

The admissions person was very kind and answered our direct questions, but there is still much we don't know. I have no idea how a nursing home operates and what we should expect. When I said you were not doing a good job, I meant that you should write a book or pamphlet containing all the information that a prospective family member or resident needs to know, such as the mystique of Medicaid and what about Medicare? I have searched libraries looking for information and there isn't much that even I can understand. Not the kind I want anyway." I might add here that this visit occurred before the advent of the internet, but I don't think the internet offers all of the type of information you will find here.

That was many years ago and he was very appreciative of how we cared for his mother. I still often think about him and his mother. I don't know why but they always stood out in my memory. I don't remember my visitor's name but he lives in my memory.

To today's reader, I can't tell you everything I know about long-term care but I hope that what I write will cause you to feel more at ease about nursing homes in general. I hope you will realize that we, in long-term care, are not the sadists everyone seems to think we are, forever depriving the residents of their dignity and privacy, and maybe killing them along the way.

And so, let us begin to learn about long-term care.

Chapter Two

The Nursing Home in Society

I invested a good part of my life in long-term care taking care of the elderly, the infirm and the just plain crazy. I touched many peoples' lives and always for the better, I hope. But I have always known the horrid connotation of the words *nursing home*. I hurt all those years knowing that our industry's reputation was close to or worse than a leper colony or slaughter house. My mother even surrendered to this way of thinking when we were both invited to an upscale cocktail party at the local country club. She sidled up to me and whispered, "Can't you tell them that you're a hospital administrator rather than a nursing home administrator?" I smiled at her and said, "No way." She was not happy. Neither was I.

What really is it that causes nursing homes to be so reviled? For the most part, nursing homes are hated.

Could it be all the bad media stories? Have you ever read a positively slanted media story regarding nursing homes? Or could it be that we all fear the late "golden years" and death? Is a nursing home the last stop before the grim reaper comes to call? A visit to a nursing home can bring these fears to the surface because we know it may not be that long until we are in the same situation. The attorneys, spread across the country, that advertise to bring you a reward for your loved one's physical and mental *anguish* suffered at the hands of the unscrupulous nursing home don't help a bit. They create fear in a population that believes everything an attorney says is correct. We all know attorneys can twist the facts, and the nursing-home-raider attorney is a master of this so-called talent. We forget that these attorneys are not doing what they do for your loved one that is or was in a nursing home; they are doing it for themselves, and they make a lot of money. The long-term care industry generally settled out of court as they were afraid of juries. Why? The jury members probably all hate nursing homes too, and we were afraid we wouldn't get a fair decision. Today, the tide is turning and the industry is winning jury trials when warranted. It's about time!

I do not intend to change the minds of those who wish all nursing homes would be closed down. But then, what if they were? I have heard horrific tales from family members who could no longer care for their loved one. The sleepless nights hoping the patient would not leave the bed and wander into the night, maybe to become forever lost. The day-to-day care for those who may require feeding or who are incontinent. The terrible changes in the personality that Alzheimer's can bring. Who among us would not be hurt when our own mother forgets our name, the name she gave you? Do you believe you could exist and have some semblance of a life if you were the sole caregiver for such a person? I don't care if this person is your mother. The constant care doesn't take long to make the caregiver desperate. Here is where those "awful" nursing homes can come to the rescue. The caregiver suffers from terrible guilt but knows there is nothing left to do but search for a good nursing home. What if there were no long-term care facilities? In today's time, there are generally two income-earners in a household. Who is going to stay with Momma and give the constant care? Well, you can advertise for someone to come in and stay with her. Lots of luck with this. Number one; it is very expensive. Number two; it is difficult to find someone dependable and number three; the stories of caregivers abusing the patient and even stealing are rampant. It even happened in my family. My father hired a nice appearing lady to go grocery shopping and drive him around on errands. It's too bad that he also gave her his checkbook. Since he was blind, he had no idea of what checks he was signing. She made away with thousands of dollars. You would be one of the few exceptions if you made this work.

And so I conclude that the nursing facility is a necessary part of society, particularly with our ever-increasing aged population. What would we do without them?

I think this is a good time to point out that, yes; there are still poorly-performing nursing homes. They're becoming fewer and fewer though due to the extremely rigid regulations, both state and federal, that nursing homes must obey today to the letter. The long-term care industry is the most regulated industry in the country. It was once nuclear energy that was the most regulated, but they fell out of the number one spot a long time ago.

I remember visiting my grandfather in a nursing home that was a big Midwestern Victorian house on a corner. Beds were everywhere, lined up in the living room and the dining room with three or four to each bedroom. The smell of urine was incredibly strong, clinging to your clothing and hair. Upon leaving, the bathroom was the first stop at home for a good bath, shampoo, and change of clothes. There were few or no regulations then. Even now, in some nursing facilities, you can smell urine. That's a sign of poor management because it doesn't have to happen. Occasionally, you may smell what we call a *transient odor* occurring when an incontinent resident is being cleaned and changed, but that is to be expected.

It is my hope that when the hospital discharge planner tells you that you must find a nursing home for your loved one, this effort of mine will help you. We'll begin with how to tour prospective skilled nursing homes.

Chapter Three

Touring Nursing Homes

Let's do a little story, a vignette in which I will take my friend, Theresa, on two tours of nursing facilities. Her mother is coming out of the hospital very soon and long-term care placement will be necessary for her. It has been determined that Theresa's mom will be eligible for Medicare coverage because of having had extensive surgery that will require daily wound-care and later, daily therapy. It seems as though she has developed two or three decubitus ulcers while in the hospital for the surgery which will require treatment to heal. This is definitely not an unusual occurrence. It is my belief that most hospital nurses have forgotten what they learned in Nursing 101. The elderly and even semi-elderly, if bedridden, must be turned every two hours without fail, in hopes of preventing the bedsores that definitely can be prevented.

Theresa has been talking to people in the community and a couple of the local nursing homes have already been eliminated from her further consideration. She's now down to two facilities and the caseworker at the hospital is putting some pressure on her to find a place to admit her mother. The time has come and she just has to make a decision about a nursing home, like it or not. Mom's doctor at the hospital wouldn't recommend a facility. He went on to say that while he didn't practice in nursing homes, he knew the doctors that would be caring for her mom and he could keep track of her in that manner.

Her choices appear to be Rosewood Manor which has been around quite a while but has a good reputation and then we have Lake Pleasant which is a brand new state-of-the-art center. Both nice names. As we get into the car, I nod and say, "Ok, let's go. We're going find the best place for your mom." I had already told her the things we were going to look at in the tours. We have appointments with Admissions Directors in both centers, starting with Rosewood Manor. We pull up and park in the lot directly in front of the building. "Let's look around for a minute", I said. The lawn is trimmed and the landscaping looked well cared for. The building could stand a new coat of paint, but looked OK. There are flowers in planters on both sides of the walkway up to the double doors of the entrance. We walk through the front doors and I whisper, "Theresa, what do you smell?" "Nothing," she replied.

If we were keeping score, we would now have two plusses. The receptionist pointed out the Admissions Director's office and we went to stand in her doorway. She was on the phone, but immediately hung up, and we did the introductions. Her name was Annette. She offered us chairs and did we want a soft drink? "How about a cup of coffee?" We declined her kind offers and told her that we would like to inquire as to the availability of beds, the financial picture regarding admissions, and take a tour of the building. The discharge planner at the hospital had already faxed over the paperwork on Theresa's mom so Annette was familiar with the case and the required care. After assuring us that a bed was available and that Mom would be covered by Medicare, she briefly described the costs covered by Medicare, and what the costs would be for a private-paying resident should she stay in the center after the Medicare coverage expired. She then asked our preference for a beginning point and I said, "Let's start with a tour." If we didn't like what we saw on the tour, there would be no sense in wasting our time and taking up the Admission Director's time as well. "Before we go, we'd like to see your last two annual surveys from the state and any other surveys you might have had in the last two years." She willingly complied and handed us the survey copies that she had waiting in her desk. There were deficiencies; five or six of them but they were insignificant and really none of them pertained to patient care. The maintenance man was short one required fire drill for the year and the surveyors found some grease buildup on the bottom of cookware in the kitchen and the rest of the deficiencies were just as trivial. Theresa and I were both pleased.

A deficiency-free survey is almost unheard of. I've been very fortunate to have had three in my facilities over the twenty-seven years. The three-and-a-half-day scrutiny by the surveyors is more than intense. They comb through charts, walk the halls talking to and observing residents (fingernail condition, clothing, etc.), they observe all resident meals, and observe many medication passes done by the nurses. The surveyors always have a private meeting with the residents so they might learn something they had not turned up on their own. It used to be that if a bed was pushed against a wall it was a deficiency, even if it was the resident's wish. This may have since changed, but I doubt it. If a resident has a bib on in the dining room, it could be a deficiency because the bib lessens the resident's dignity. I always personally thought that food spilled down a dress or shirt would have been less dignified, but then who am I to say? The surveyors leave absolutely nothing untouched. All the departments get their own intense scrutiny such as Nursing, Housekeeping, Dietary, Administration, Maintenance, Activities and Social Services.

Walking down a hall with Annette, we noted that the floors were gleaming, a little wax build-up along the edges, but perfectly clean. The walls were painted a delicate peach color, and a darker hue of peach framed the doorways of the resident rooms. We passed a well-organized nursing station and noted the licensed nursing staff busy at work. They all wore colorful scrub outfits, complete with name tags. I had already explained to my friend that nursing homes don't use the white starched uniforms anymore, and very seldom will you even see a lab coat. The reason being is that the nursing facility is a home for the residents and we try to make the centers *social models* rather than *medical models*. One of the nurses spoke to us and smiled. She said, "If you see 'Irish', tell him I've got a treat for him." Just at that moment, a large red Irish Setter padded around the corner and sat in front of us, tail a-wag, hoping for a good rub around his ears, which he promptly received. The nurse gave a biscuit to the appreciative dog and explained, "Irish is our facility pet. The residents love him and he sleeps in their rooms at night and during the day, for that matter. He takes turns with all those who want him around. He's such a special dog and I don't know what we'd do without him. The staff shares in taking care of him and we think he feels that he is one lucky dog, which he is." Another nurse spoke to Annette and said there was a call for her. I told her to go ahead that we would just wander around the center. She smiled and said that she would catch up with us.

Continuing down the hall, we almost ran into a couple

of certified nursing assistants coming out of a room. As we excused ourselves, one of the aides grinned and replied, "Don't you think a thing about that. Are you here to maybe admit someone?" We nodded, and she said, "Well, you've come to the right place. We love our residents." Where's my score card? I need to enter some more plusses.

Annette, true to her word, had re-joined us and she led Theresa and me into a vacant room with two-well made beds separated by a hospital-type cubicle curtain. The bedspreads were colorful, and the view out the window was of the front lawn. There was one bathroom shared by the occupants in this room and the adjacent room. In other words, a four person bathroom. Neither of us were too impressed by this fact. Theresa asked if they had any private rooms and Annette, the Admissions Director, professionally explained that since the resident was going to be covered by Medicare, she would have to be in a Medicare-certified bed. A Medicaid resident can go into any bed in the center as can a private paying resident, but the Medicare resident can only go into the Medicare certified bed. The two beds in the room were both Medicare certified beds. She laughed and said, "That's the government for you. They don't allow their Medicare covered patients to have a private room unless it is for a special medical reason documented by the attending physician." I nodded as I knew this to be true. (For more information regarding Medicaid and

Medicare, please see Chapter 10).

The next stop was the large dining room with a group of residents playing Bingo, a favorite game at most nursing facilities. They all looked clean and well-dressed. The Activity Director was calling the Bingo numbers, but she waved to us as we passed. We came to a large glass-framed case mounted at wheelchair height on the wall in the dining room. Posted inside were the activities and the three dining menus for the day. The menus looked quite good and reminded us of country food. The day was jam-packed with activities; all the way from arts and crafts, to current events talks, and even a reminiscence group meeting. In these meetings, the leader sets a topic such as "The Great Depression" and the residents talk about what happened to them during this time. Another good topic is "Going to School in a One-Room Schoolhouse". Next to the glass case was posted a gigantic decorated calendar that showed the activities for every day of the month. Since we were nearing Easter, it was cleverly decorated with an Easter motif complete with bunnies, eggs, baskets and flowers. We passed a conference room where a resident care plan meeting had just ended so were able to meet the department heads whose jobs touched resident care. We were particularly interested in the Dietary Manager, as Theresa's mom was somewhat of a finicky eater. She assured us that she does everything possible to make a resident content and explained that if a resident didn't like what was on the menu, a special meal could be prepared. And what about snacks? She nodded her head and said, "Nobody ever goes hungry around here. There are usually snacks during activities, and a cart loaded with goodies and fruit makes the rounds every day and at bedtime. If one of our residents should wake up hungry in the middle of the night, we have food at the nurse's station such as cereals, soup, peanut butter, graham crackers, and fruit." She went on, "I do a 'likes and dislikes' survey on every new admission and we don't have much of a weight-loss problem here because we give the residents what they want to eat. We do our best to persuade the doctors from not ordering strict medical diets, if at all possible, except for the diabetics, of course. We had a lady here last month that loved goats' milk so I stopped every morning at a grocery that carried goats' milk to be sure that I always had it on hand for her. She drank a lot of it and it cut into my food budget that I operate with, but if a resident wants something, I'll get it for them. No problem." Annette was again paged for a telephone call so she left us with the promise she'd be back as soon as she could.

As we continued down the hall, we and saw two ladies in a lively conversation sitting in a room overlooking a vegetable garden and having iced tea. We rapped on the door and asked if we could visit for a few moments with them. They seemed excited to have the company and answered all our questions to the affirmative. Did they like it here? "Oh, yes, we wouldn't think of going any place else since we can't go home." I asked, "What about the staff? Do they treat you well?" The lady on the left with a beautiful grey 'bob' haircut sweetly replied that they were very nice but she wished they didn't have to work so hard. The little lady in pink on the right nodded and echoed her friend. We thanked them for their time and they begged us to stay and maybe have supper with them. We told them of our next appointment at Lake Pleasant, and that it was time for us to leave. They looked slyly at one another and giggled, "That won't take long. We get a lot of people from that place." We said our goodbyes and left to a chorus of, "We'll see you soon! Come back and visit! Take Care!" We both felt vaguely guilty about leaving, but it was time to be thinking of the next appointment.

About this time, the Activity Director, done with her Bingo session, was walking toward us and stopped to chat. She informed us that she did a thorough assessment on every new admission. She also did her best to tailor activities that interest the most residents possible, to include as many different types of interests as she could.

She said, "We also have in-room activities for those who cannot or do not wish to join us in the dining room where most of our activities take place. If the resident likes to knit, read, work on crossword puzzles, even color or draw, we provide all the necessary materials in a basket for their room. Naturally, we want our residents to get out of their room if they can, make friends and enjoy the activities and outings we provide. Our outings generally happen once or twice a month and we go to a mall, out to lunch, and maybe to the lake for fishing and a picnic. We always let our residents suggest where they would like to go."

It was nearing our time to leave. We said our goodbyes and thanked Annette for being so helpful and informative. She handed us several pamphlets loaded with facts and figures about the center and Medicare. She waved to us as we left the center.

After a short ride across town, we arrived, right on time, at an absolutely gorgeous new facility. The landscaping was lush. There was a gazebo and even an exercise trail for the residents through the extensive grassy grounds with many shade trees and benches. The facility was in the process of filling to its capacity of 120 beds and they were filling those beds as fast as they could so as to keep the Administrator's financial bottom line continually rising out of the red. We entered the tall, elegant glass front doors and found ourselves in a large lobby. It had the decorator's stamp all over everything, even the comfy new furniture. There were no residents in the lobby. Good so far, but deep down, I knew what we would probably find. I wondered why there were no residents taking advantage of this lovely room.

We were directed to the Admission Coordinator's office. To our dismay, there were two couples ahead of us. The flustered admissions person said that she was running late and it would probably be another forty minutes until she could speak with us. She told us to feel free to look around which suited me to a tee. We walked down the brightly lit hall and peered into the beautiful unoccupied rooms, some semi-private and some private. The beds were carefully made and everything was brand-spanking new. The decorator stamp was in the resident rooms as well. Both of us looked at each other and nodded but I wasn't ready to give the approval nod, not by a long shot. We proceeded on down the hall and came to a unit where some of the newly-admitted residents lived. Nobody stopped us or asked if we needed help. Suddenly, I got a good strong whiff. Urine. Old urine. I am an experienced urine connoisseur and can tell you if it is fresh or approximately how old it is in one sniff. I have other talents but this is one of my lesser known abilities. We saw piles of dirty linen thrown on the floor in the rooms and bathrooms (a strict nursing no-no because of infection control) and I was quite positive that these soiled sheets contained their share of feces and urine. Residents all in wheelchairs were lined up in the hall across from the nursing station. They stared blankly ahead and were paid very little attention by anyone. They had no stimulation, no music. Nothing. Automatically, I checked the residents' fingernails and they were all filthy, even broken and torn. It appeared, to my experienced eye, that some of them had not been bathed in a while and their hair was hanging in greasy strands. Their clothing, for the most part, was stained with what was eaten for lunch that day, and maybe breakfast as well. If I cared to, I probably could have figured out the day's menu in detail just by the clothing. We passed a large, but vacant activities room. I saw the Activity Director in her glass-walled office working on charts rather than keeping her residents busy and happy. While it is very true that charting is a necessary evil, it should take place either before or after the activities for the day. We continued on to a large dining room that was exquisitely decorated and had massive arrangements of silk flowers in all the right places. The room didn't smell right. I wandered around to the cart room outside the kitchen door and there were piles of badly soiled dishes stacked up and a large basin full of the scrapings from the plates. There were many, many dishes from lunch and it was nearing 4 p.m. I wondered what they would use for supper, probably paper plates. Further on, we noted a rather surly housekeeper mopping the floor grumbling to herself as we passed by. As was my habit, I checked the color of the water in her mop bucket. It was as I expected, filthy black and it had not been changed according to any infection control policy I ever heard of.

I stopped in a small alcove, turned to Theresa and said, "Have you seen enough?"

"Oh, hell yes. Let's get outta here."

I explained to her in the car that I had opened four new centers and that there are pitfalls galore in a new opening (as we witnessed). The department heads frequently turn over twice in the first year. The licensed nursing staff doesn't know the aides and nothing has jelled yet. Add this to the company's constantly haranguing the administrator to fill up the beds faster and faster. In my four new center openings, I filled each in 90 days. It was extremely difficult, to say the very least and quite similar to herding a passel of cats. We always passed our initial surveys from the state with very few deficiencies, due only to the hardest work by everyone. An administrator in this sort of situation has to be well-experienced and a pretty fair leader, walking the halls constantly looking for problems that must be solved, and be fortunate enough to have a good department heads. We muddled through, however, and I was always lucky enough to be able to grade the patient care with a 'B' during the opening. After we were full at the capacity of 120 residents, things calmed down and we were ready to fine-tune all systems. A nursing center is full of systems. If they are all in place, everything runs smoothly. However, if one or two break down, you've got a 'tiger' on your hands. You've got to recognize the tiger stripes early on before the animal attacks and get the problem solved so that the system will be up and operating once again.

Theresa chose Rosewood Manor, thinking that her mother would be happy there. She still was not happy about having to share a toilet and sink with three other people but thought that her mother could adjust. She was already planning on personalizing her mother's room with treasures brought from home and I believe Theresa now felt a lot better about her mother coming out of the hospital. Her mom was admitted a couple of days later and when I last heard, she was as happy as a clam and even gaining weight.

Chapter Four

Selecting the Right Nursing Center

The following is a list of some of the things you should look for or question. The list is in no particular order as to importance. Everything is important when deciding which is the right facility for you or your loved one. Please remember we are speaking of a skilled nursing center or SNF.

* Ease of making the initial appointment by telephone.

* Treatment upon arrival. Were you welcomed and escorted or politely directed to the Admission Coordinator's office?

* What do you smell? Odors are generally worse early in the morning. If you detect stale urine odors after ten a.m., just imagine what they smelled like at seven a.m. Remember, nursing homes should not have

odors except for the occasional transient odor.

* Experience with Admissions Coordinator. Good? Or were you not impressed?

* Did you look at the latest state survey? How many deficiencies total? How many in patient care? Did the deficiencies in patient care appear serious? Do not hesitate to ask questions regarding the deficiencies. If you are not satisfied with what the Admissions Director tells you, please ask to see the administrator and director of nursing.

* What are the Private and Semi-private rates? How do they compare with other centers? What is included in the rates?

* Were you given handouts regarding the center? Were they helpful?

* Were you given information on Medicaid and Medicare?

* Does the center have a VA contract?

* What is the overall appearance of the center (inside and outside)?

* Cleanliness. Shining floors? (Don't worry. Nursing facilities use non-skid wax.) Look in the corners.

Look for dust on furniture, windowsills and under beds. Check the condition of the paint. Look at the linen. Are the sheets gray and thin? What about the towels? Are they dingy and thin?

* Appearance of rooms. Is there a TV or will you have to bring one? What about cable? Is it supplied or do you have to pay for it? Can rooms be personalized with items from home? Is there a telephone? If not, can one be installed?

* Appearance of the bathrooms. Odor? Condition of floors? How many will have to share one bathroom? Would you feel comfortable using the bathroom?

* How many beds are in the center? How many are Medicare certified?

* Appearance of residents. Note hair, clothing (are they dressed appropriately and are they clean?), and fingernails. Greasy hair, food-stained clothing and dirty ragged fingernails are dead giveaways regarding poor overall patient care.

* Food issues? Did you hear any complaints? Were you able to observe a meal? Did the food look attractive and well-prepared? Was the day's menu posted? Was the menu posted at a level where a wheelchair bound resident could see it? Were all the residents at a table served together or did one or two

have to wait for their meals while watching their table partners eat?

* Were you able to meet the administrator and director of nursing? What were your feelings? Did they appear open and easy to talk to? If you wish to speak to either of them, is it necessary to make an appointment?

* Overall staff friendliness. Did they look you in the eye? Smile? Speak to you? How were they dressed? Were they neat and clean?

* How many physicians practice at the center? Will you be able to choose among them?

* Is there an Alzheimer's Unit or a Specialized Unit? (When touring this unit use all the above suggestions to rate it as well as the center, in general). What are the residents doing during your visit? Are they lined up in a hall with nothing to do or are they engaged in some sort of activity? Do all "behavior problem" residents live on this unit or are they mixed throughout the center?

* Does the center have a dentist that will see the residents, and also act as consultant?

* Is there an activities schedule posted both in the main part of the facility and also in the Alzheimer's

Unit? Do the activities appear varied and sound like they might be fun?

* Visit the therapy department. Do they have many rehab residents? Do they offer the three therapies: Physical, Occupational and Speech? If the therapists are part time make sure that their schedule will agree with your loved one's needs in the case therapy has been ordered by the physician.

* Look at staffing particularly in the nursing department. Ask the administrator or director of nursing what the staffing ratio is. If you don't understand, ask them to give you examples. The requirements vary by state. (I have given you the formula for correctly figuring the correct nursing staff numbers in another part of this book - under Nursing Staff. Chapter 7.)

* What hospitals does the center have transfer agreements with?

* If you are located on a coastline or any other place of possible danger, ask to see the disaster plan and question as to where the residents will be evacuated if this becomes necessary. Remember, you don't have to be in a hurricanes' favorite path or in tornado alley, there could be a large chemical spill, a fire, train derailment. All sorts of things can happen and there needs to be a well-thought-out plan.

* I would ask to see their fire drill log.

* Is the latest regulatory agency survey posted where it can be easily seen? Is information on Medicare and Medicaid posted there as well?

* Has the Admission's Coordinator thoroughly explained the process of laundering resident clothing? She should tell you that every piece of clothing must be clearly marked with the resident's name (not where it can be seen by the public) with laundry pens....only permanent ink pens designed for laundry marking. For black socks, they make white marking pens. She should also tell you that all items of clothing (and other personal items) must be entered on the resident inventory sheet, which is usually located in the resident's chart. I hope she will tell you that it is not necessary to bring all of a person's clothing to the facility. The facility has no place to store a complete wardrobe. A few changes will be sufficient. Every time you bring in new items or remove items, the inventory sheet must indicate this activity. Please help the staff keep the inventory sheets accurate. Lost clothing is common in most centers but it shouldn't have to be if the family members label every item that is brought into the center. This problem is mentioned again later.

* Is it possible for you to attend a resident council

meeting? You would have to be invited by the residents but it might be worth your while asking.

* Does the center have a way of marking eye glasses and dentures? Please make sure this happens. I've seen boxes at nurses stations filled with lost glasses and no way to find the proper owner.

* Is there a store for personal items, stamps, candy, etc. on the premises?

* Did you see a beauty shop? How many times a week does the hairdresser come? Does she/he cut men's hair too? How do you make an appointment? And how much are the various services?

* Does the center have a newsletter? How often it is published?

* Are there outside patios with decent furniture for visiting families and friends? Some centers have a swing set and toys for visiting children.

Most of these items are addressed in different areas of this book but it is always handy to have a check list when visiting nursing homes.

* If your resident must be transported for an outside physician appointment or to a dentist, please plan on taking care of this yourself. If the center does not

employ a person to accompany residents to appointments, a nursing assistant will have to be taken away from her work on the floor to take the resident. Since this assistant is counted into the staffing ratio, it is not right to remove her from the floor as it cuts into the care time for the other residents. Ask how the center handles these outside appointments.

* Ask about the set up the facility has for the Patient Trust Fund. This is a way that your resident can have money for a hair cut or a Coke without having to keep money in their room, which might be stolen either by staff members or other residents. How often will they send statements to you?

The previous suggestions should serve you well. Never be shy about asking a lot of questions when you visit. You probably won't find a perfect center like Rosewood Manor (I hope you do) but there are quite a few Lake Pleasants out there, old and new.

Chapter Five

The Social Model of the Nursing Home

There has been a wind of change blowing through the long-term care industry. Years ago, we did all we could to emulate the hospitals. Our nurses wore the starched whites with their school nursing cap and pin. Everything ran by a prescribed routine that generally always favored the facility. Woe be unto the one who thought relaxing the system would be of more benefit to our patients (we called them patients in the old days but as the change began to take place, the term 'resident' took the place of 'patient'). Our kitchens produced as many special diets as the hospital kitchens. These special diets were never well-received by the patients and weight loss abounded, which caused the physicians to order more and more dietary supplements such as Ensure. At one time, back in the medical model dark-ages, I was spending far more for Ensure than I was for all nursing supplies.

Allow a pet in the center? Never! It was well known that dogs and cats carried massive amounts of pathogens that might cause big trouble in our "near sterile" environment. I have to giggle when I remember how everyone gasped when we heard of an administrator that ran several Clydesdale horses through the halls of an east Georgia facility. The residents loved the parade, the housekeepers did not and neither did the director of nursing.

We allowed our patients to eat in their beds or in their rooms. (We all had large roach populations in the resident rooms). It was easier than dragging over 100 people to the dining room at the same time. This didn't help the patients' social skills at all, but it helped a great deal in the continued institutionalization of the patients. Even today in the centers that have adopted the social model there is some institutionalization in residents though we work diligently to keep this from occurring. In those "olden" days, the routine was "King" and I always thought it was a way to get the most work out of the fewest nursing staff members. The patients were gotten up at more or less the same time every morning and some of them far too early, just for the staff convenience. The daily agenda for the residents never changed. It was breakfast, lunch, Bingo, supper and then bed, the same thing day in and day out. I remember when I was a director of nursing in southwest Georgia (and yes, I wore the starched whites, the pin and the school nursing cap), the administrator and I decided to have a wine and cheese party for the patients who had permission from the doctors for a bit of alcohol from time to time. The nursing home was located in a tiny village of no more than 100 people (the census of the nursing home was larger than the population) but this tiny dot on the map boasted three churches. The party was a huge success and we even were able to talk a couple of the patients into dancing. Come Sunday morning, we were lambasted from the pulpits of all three churches and even had visits from angry villagers who spoke of our corrupting their sacred elderly. Having adult fun was not at the top of the list for their elderly, but they very much approved of the annual Easter egg hunts. It was both ludicrous and sad to see our elderly (those who could walk) stumbling through the field across the street, basket in hand, looking for Easter eggs. Talk about deprivation of dignity! Oh well, it was a break in the deadly monotony of their days.

Slowly, we began to change. Patients became residents; the severe special diets eased and were used only when absolutely necessary. Patients' Rights (now called Residents' Rights) had always been with us but now we honored them ever more closely. If a diabetic didn't want his sugar-free dessert but wanted a piece of that nice chocolate cake his neighbor was eating, all efforts would be made to inform him of the possible consequences of eating the cake. If he insisted, he would have his yummy piece of chocolate cake. Of course the nurse would be notified, it would be charted, the resident would be monitored and even the doctor would be notified if the resident was a brittle diabetic.

It was slow, but as we changed, we began to see happier residents and even fewer hospitalizations in some cases. We all didn't change at the same pace and there were a few problems but most of us in the industry wanted the change, so eventually it happened. Some of us from my company were allowed to attend a four-day conference in Chicago on how to achieve the social model nursing home atmosphere. We learned new things to try to get more into the social model, and came back to the nursing facility, full of excitement. We had plans to implement so many great changes but to our dismay, our company would not allow any extra money so we did it ourselves. It wasn't hard and the staff bonded even more working to employ more and more changes.

Those centers that have changed their focus from *medical* model to *social* model are quite adept at providing fun activities for their residents and making the resident their number one priority in how the nursing home is run. Now a resident doesn't have to get out of bed at the crack of dawn to satisfy the aide's schedule and there are lots of parties. There are some centers that have gone so far as to allow the residents to have their room cleaned at a time most convenient for them. Some centers even attempt to serve meals when the resident wishes. This is very difficult with the state and federal regulations about how many hours can be between the dinner and breakfast meals and to cater to everyone's time preference is almost impossible.

It is not known how many centers have adopted this social model. It is not difficult to do. It just takes changing old ideas into new and fresh ideas.

These social-model centers never rotate their nurses and certified nursing assistants from assignment to assignment, or hall to hall. It is so important that the residents keep the same staff as it gives the residents and the nursing staff stability because they come to know each other so well. The aides become very involved with their long term residents who, for the most part, are their friends. No, not all are friends but if we, as management, see a problem between a member of the nursing staff and a resident, all is done to adjust the staff to make everyone happy. And no, it doesn't always work. I remember a paraplegic lady in her 40s that got about with a motorized wheelchair. This lady was the most demanding resident I have ever known. She had her very own schedule involving sleeping late and wanting to get up at the same time that the aides were serving lunch in the dining room. Many times the ill and disabled can be very demanding because they desperately must have at least a little control over their lives. So understandable, but the aides that ran a pretty tight schedule and were trying to please everyone just couldn't adapt to her personal schedule. Somehow, they handled it but not without many complaints from the resident who was a frequent visitor in my office with her motorized wheelchair. Her complaints began at 12:30 p.m. and lasted a half hour every day. I just naturally cleared my work to be ready for her. (I did what I could with the staff trying to adjust schedules but there was no hope.) I did my best with the resident but she brushed aside my best efforts and called her daughter. The daughter was an ally of mine as she understood her mother very well. The resident not only had to deal with her paraplegia, she had very serious lung problems that caused her to be hospitalized many times. Most of the time she was on oxygen, but she was a dedicated smoker as well. She had a wire contraption that fit on her wheelchair to hold her cigarette of the moment. She required a person to place the cigarette in the holder and also to light the cigarette. It truly was never-ending. She had another love besides her cigarettes and that was alcohol. Occasionally, she would leave the facility without checking out and drive her wheelchair up the streets to her favorite bar. Her missing from the center was always a major event but we knew where to find her. She even was pulled over by the police several times in her wheelchair and she thought this to be hilarious. She loved to drive over a major highway to a

7-11 convenience store for beer. Though she was very difficult to care for, we still loved her and grieved when she passed away during an emphysema attack while hospitalized.

There are generally several halls in a nursing center and a newly admitted person may choose whichever available bed they want with the exception of the Medicare resident having to occupy a Medicare certified bed. Beyond this, the resident who is moderately to severely demented, or an Alzheimer's victim, generally functions at a higher level in the Alzheimer's unit, if one is available.

Each hall has 'block parties' and the aides and nurses put on real wing-dings for their residents. Every staff member (and sometimes family members) brings a dish; there are decorations and even music for dancing. Some halls have outdoor areas and if so, the residents might choose to have BBQs on the patio with hamburgers, potato salad, and watermelon. It is not unusual for one hall to invite the entire facility to their block party. The residents love these parties and look forward to the next one.

I have always believed that nursing homes should have animals. My last facility boasted a wild bird aviary that contained approximately 30 birds. They made their nests, laid their eggs and had their young, all while being watched by the residents. They loved the birds.

Then there was Fifi, the gentleman guinea pig that preferred to be a lady named Fifi. There were 2 ferrets that the residents took care of. Add a cat or maybe two and residents' dogs and we usually had quite a menagerie. Everyone loved this except the director of housekeeping but we were very careful to keep cleanliness in mind when caring and playing with the animals.

In keeping with our new social model, I suggested at one of our monthly Florida Health Care Association meetings, attended by administrators and sometimes directors of nursing from twelve or fifteen centers, that we have a beauty pageant annually for our residents. I outlined the program for them and the association voted unanimously to do the first pageant. How I envisioned this was that in April, a large pageant would be held in each of the separate facilities to elect a "Ms. (name of the nursing home)". The dining room would be decorated with ferns and flowers. The volunteer contestants would be dressed in long gowns, have their hair, makeup and nails done, and wear nice jewelry donated by family members or staff. Each lady would be given a florist-made corsage to wear. All family members and the public were invited to attend and all available chairs were arranged theater-style. As each visitor came in to be seated, he or she would be given a program that contained the contestants' biographies. A volunteer would play old love songs softly on the piano as the pageant began. As the music played, each lady was escorted down the center aisle by a volunteer who owned a tuxedo. The Master of Ceremonies would announce the lady's name and give a brief biography. All contestants sat in a semi-circle facing the audience. When all the contestants were seated, the MC would tell the ladies that he would be asking each one of them prewritten questions and for them to please speak loudly when answering. He would hold the microphone for each one of them as they answered the questions. There was a panel of 4 judges (in my case, the local mayor, a newspaper reporter, a teacher, and a government social worker). Each would make notes as to how the contestants looked and how they answered the questions. Were they humorous? Their personalities counted along with several other attributes. Finally the big moment would arrive. The votes were counted and the winner was announced. She would stand (if possible) to receive a bouquet of long stemmed red roses and a ribbon sash imprinted with Ms._____ (whatever nursing home) and a plaque proclaiming her win would be presented as soon as it could be engraved with her name. Following the pageant, a buffet reception was held for all.

A month later, the grand pageant would be held and all the winners from each facility would be sporting a sash that indicated the Ms. and what nursing home she was from. This event could be held in any large place. I have had pageants in college theaters, the United

States Naval Museum at the Pensacola Naval Air Station with the Blue Angel jet planes hanging high overhead (the ladies were escorted by Marines in dress uniform), and once even in a downtown theater. From the contestants, the grand winner was chosen who received nice prizes donated by local merchants, another bouquet of long-stemmed red roses, a tiara, and a beautiful framed proclamation of her being named "Ms. Florida Health Care Association."

Everyone loved the pageants. They were a lot of work for everyone, but seeing the beaming faces of the beautiful ladies in their gowns and splendor made it so worth while and was guaranteed to bring a tear of joy.

Chapter Six

Common Problems in the Nursing Home

No matter what we do, no matter how hard we try, there are things that just happen.

LOST CLOTHING

I know I've mentioned this before but, oh, what a problem! We require families to clearly label every item of the residents' clothing whether or not the facility does the laundry. (Families have the choice of doing their resident's laundry.) Then why do so many clothing items get lost? Where do they go?

Sometimes, family members bring in new clothes that aren't labeled and are not entered on the belongings inventory kept in the resident's chart. The nursing staff can be lax in keeping the inventory sheets up. It's a job that takes time, and sometimes there just isn't enough time and they hate to do it. Family members should check the inventory sheets frequently to make sure they are current and complete.

Another reason is that even though a family may have placed a sign in the room with big red, block letters reading, "FAMILY DOES LAUNDRY", the, aide out of habit, puts the soiled item in the facility laundry. This happens because the aide is in a hurry and doesn't think about that big red lettered sign on the clothes hamper that was brought from home. When the clothing item comes back from the laundry, it might and it might not reach the right closet, even though it is labeled. I couldn't dare guess how many meetings I've had with the nursing and laundry people on this problem, mostly to no avail. The laundry always has piles of unlabeled clothing items and, occasionally, they put them out on racks so residents and family members might find lost items. Black socks were always to first to go missing because of the problem in labeling. Once, I hired a seamstress to sew labels into every item of residents' clothing. I wore out three seamstresses, and at the end, this didn't work either, mainly because of clothing items continually brought in by family members that were not labeled and not placed on the inventory sheet.

I've tried system after system and none were very successful. Another factor that comes into play is the confused little lady resident who likes to go "shopping" in the various closets taking what she likes back to her own closet. About every two to three weeks the aides have to go through all the closets and send the items back to the proper owner. Laundry is a difficult problem not helped by family members bringing in too many clothes that just are not necessary.

I would bet that half of the complaints I received in over a quarter century as an administrator and regional manager of nursing homes were about missing items, clothing in particular.

LOST JEWELRY

Your loved one does not need his or her jewelry collection with them at the nursing home. Valuables must be left at home or placed in the safe in the front office of the nursing home if this service is offered. Even though most family members comply with this, they might elect to leave the thin, worn wedding band on their mother or father. We do our best to protect this ring, but residents will frequently take rings and bracelets off, put them on the bedside table, and the items can easily fall into the waste basket, or a confused "shopper" may decide she needed more jewelry. Another thing that can happen is that the resident may be experiencing a weight loss and the wedding band slips off the finger, goes to the laundry with the bedding, and is forever lost. That is a very sad thing for everyone.

LOST DENTURES, GLASSES, AND HEARING AIDES

Yes, I know I'm repeating myself. It us a huge problem for all involved: Residents frequently take their dentures, hearing aid or glasses and lay them on the bedside table. Though there are containers for the residents' use, many forget to use them and they end up in the laundry or the trash. Sometimes the laundry will retrieve items but unless the resident's name is etched on the item, even the dentures, we have little way of finding the proper owner. The dentures and hearing aids have multiple-sided problems in that residents sometimes just throw them away because they no longer fit. Dentures and wearing the hearing aide can be uncomfortable, and the resident doesn't want to tell the family member so it would be stated by the resident that the item in question just disappeared. This wasn't a good idea for the hapless resident because now she has to endure, at the facility's expense, dental trips for new dentures or refitting of a hearing aid that she didn't want in the first place. Were they on the inventory sheets? Hardly ever. Same with eyeglasses. While we were usually able to keep track of all items that we knew about, those that were on the inventory sheet and labeled with the resident name, other non-labeled items appeared and were promptly lost. We always had a box of eyeglasses that couldn't be identified.

I can't resist this little tale about a set of lost dentures. When working as a director of nursing, I passed through the facility dining room and saw a pair of dentures sitting all alone on top of the piano. I made a mental note to stop and get them when I returned from my errand but when I came back, they were gone. I figured that another staff member had picked them up so I went about my business. Suddenly, there was laughing emanating from the drug room behind one of the nurses' stations. I went to the door wondering what was so funny and the nurses told me they had just seen a gentleman resident with TWO sets of dentures in his mouth. They had removed the set I had seen on the piano but I wished I could have seen how in the world he got two sets into his mouth. And no, the piano dentures never did find their home.

THE LACK OF STORAGE

Another huge problem. In my many centers, we never had adequate storage for the items we needed to keep on hand such as disaster supplies, etc. It gets much worse when families come in with resident outfits for an entire year. The closet runs out of space after the first four outfits are hung. Some have even left suitcases for us to store. We informed them that we had no storage but they evidently didn't believe us. What we had to do was go into town and rent storage units. In my last center we had five large rental units. Those families who brought in seasonal clothing hardly ever took them home when the season changed. Telephone calls didn't do much good, as our problem seemed to be the least of their problems.

We always encouraged family members and residents to decorate their room space so as to make the resident feel more "at home". Some took it too literally and brought overstuffed furniture, desks, and tables; all for a semi-private room that was none too big to begin with. Mostly, they had to turn around and take it all home because there was no room in which to stand. A clear walkway must be kept for resident safety in walking, in the case of an emergency, and also for paramedics to load the very ill resident for transport to the hospital. They also brought teddy bears, stuffed rabbits, pictures, you name it, to the extreme and frequently it was so cluttered that the housekeepers could not clean. Then I had to be the bad guy to tell the resident and the family that a lot of it had to go home in order for us to clean properly.

This is probably a good time to tell you that in some areas of the country, TVs and radios might be quarantined in sealed bags by the facility for a week. In areas that have a large roach population such as

Florida and the Deep South, you will find this very common. We all know that roaches love the warm wires inside of the TV's and radios and our maintenance department had taken as many as 250 out of a radio. Speaking of unwanted "critters", candy, as well as all food items absolutely must be contained in a "snap top" plastic box. Nursing home residents love to have "munchies" at the bedside and why shouldn't they? These items must be properly stored if they are to be in the room. In the past, I have told my nursing staff to throw away every item that is not properly contained, even fruit. People yelled and screamed about this, but I didn't care. I had seen roach infestations of the worst kind in my career and I didn't want to see another one.

When a resident passes on, the furniture in his or her room may be badly soiled or stained. Family members don't like to deal with things like this, so we become responsible for taking it to the dump even though we have no truck to haul it with. On one occasion a family member, from out of town, called and told me that she would come and get her deceased mother's antique desk and the urn containing her mother's beloved pet's ashes. I put the desk in my office since I didn't have anyplace else to keep it safe and I set Fido's ashes on top. There they sat for six months and nobody ever showed up to take them home. I gave the desk away but I don't remember what happened to Fido. However, I do know that I had some superstitious housekeepers because they never dusted Fido's urn when they cleaned my office in the six months he kept me company.

FALLS

There was a very funny novel many years ago, entitled "The House of God". I have forgotten who wrote it but it was about a group of interns working in a Brooklyn hospital with a rather bizarre head resident. It was a hilarious book but parts of it about the nursing home elderly were cruel and unfortunate, but very funny. Every time a nursing home resident was brought into the emergency room with their myriad illnesses, both imagined and real, he or she was labeled a GOMER which stood for "Get out of my Emergency Room". In the front of the book are a set of "laws" that the head resident believed in. One of them was "GOMERS GO TO GROUND". Though the label of GOMER is very unkind, the GROUND part is quite accurate.

When people grow older, they become less and less steady on their feet. Add to this a dimming of the vision and a hearing loss and we've contributed a lot to the problem of falls. At one time, we used bedside rails for the bed bound residents but the state, in its infinite wisdom, said there were too many injuries resulting from people trying to climb over or through the bed-rails. We also used to use soft restraints for the residents, generally confused, who fell continuously. The state took these away even before they got to the side rails. I asked a state surveyor why take them all away when everyone knows more falls will occur. The surveyor just smiled and said, "It is the resident's right to fall." I couldn't believe my ears but not too long after, we had to remove every restraint in the building much to the dismay of the families and staff. I had call, after call and visit after visit from irate family members who eventually started a letter writing campaign to the state, all to no avail. And yes, the number of falls increased dramatically. We had many fractures. They were mostly hip fractures and also big bruises that looked as if the resident had been beaten. It was awful, but the rate of falls suddenly began to decline. We never figured out quite why but it was most likely that the staff members were watching the residents more closely. I just don't know. You cannot watch an entire population of a 120-bed facility all the time. It just isn't possible. There are going to be falls and the nursing facility has no choice but to soak up the blame. The people that fall in the facility will fall at home too and probably on a more frequent basis. To help avoid falls, the nursing facility uses non-skid floor wax and has wheelchair alarms that sound off when a resident attempts to stand. We don't allow throw rugs and are constantly looking for things that can cause falls such as inappropriate shoes. Every fall is care-planned, graphed, and investigated to find the cause. We even had to report every fall to the home office of our company. While my facilities did fairly well in this field, there was always room for improvement.

THE CONFUSED RESIDENT

As I said before, a confused resident might go "shopping" in another resident's closet. He or she may see something on a bedside table that is interesting and then it is no longer there. That Hershey bar that was being saved for bedtime? Where did it go? For the most part, we know who our "pack rats" are and we do our best to return the purloined items before they are missed.

I had a resident a long time ago that absolutely stunk. No other word for it. We couldn't even put another resident in the same room with her. She adamantly refused all bathing and any change of clothing as well. We had learned to stand clear when Maggie came down the hall so as to not catch the full stench of her. The state surveyors wanted to know why we hadn't done something about this and I informed them that whatever we did would be a violation of her resident rights. They nodded and changed the subject. Finally, we began noticing another smell in her room that wafted down the hallway. It reminded us of rotting garbage. I was working one Sunday as the RN supervisor because we had had a call-in. I didn't mind though since it gave me a chance to put on my whites again, complete with school pin and cap. (This was long before the days of the colorful scrubs and the disdaining of the white uniform and cap, and I might add, well polished white shoes.) While standing at the nurses' station, I was granted a particularly pungent whiff of Maggie and the nurses were complaining that the odor was worsening in her room. It seemed centered around her constantly locked foot locker. I decided that the time had come, and not a moment too soon, for me to take Maggie in hand; resident rights or not. I told the nurses to bring some clean clothes to the station. I told the maintenance person on duty to break the lock on Maggie's foot locker and see what was in there that was so odiferous. We then rounded Maggie up and several male orderlies bodily carried her to the shower where I was waiting. My cap was off as were my shoes. My sleeves and pant legs were rolled up as far as they would go. I was ready for Maggie, who arrived in the shower room screaming and kicking. The men held her down in the shower chair while I undressed her and scrubbed her from one end to the other with Maggie calling me every foul name she had ever heard. (I thought some of them were rather colorful). Finally, it was all over and we somehow controlled her flailing limbs enough to get her dressed. The maintenance person was waiting for me as I stumbled out of the steamy shower. He beckoned me to come with him. On entering Maggie's room, the smell of horrible decay was rampant as well as nauseating. I didn't want to look in the foot locker but

I did. It was full of unidentifiable food covered with mold and maggots at their feast. I told him to get it out back and do what he had to do. Burn it, bury it; I didn't care as long as it was gone.

Maggie always ate in her room (thank God, because of her stench) and what she didn't eat, she stored in her foot locker in case she got hungry. Maggie was not a happy camper but I wasn't either. At least the combined odors of Maggie and her foot locker had been taken care of for the time being.

I took some heat over the "Maggie Problem", mainly from one of the nurses. She said, "It was just plain wrong." Maybe it was. I had certainly violated her rights in forcing a shower on her and disposing of her property. It reminded me of the far more serious old-time story in my college ethics class where a wagon train in the old west had eluded a band of Indians passing single file along the cliff high above. Suddenly, an infant in a wagon began to wail. The mother promptly smothered her baby and the Indians passed them by. She chose to kill her child so the people in the wagon train could live. Was she right? Was she wrong? I know this story is an old saw but sometimes you cannot tell what is right and what is wrong. I would still give Maggie a bath today and I still would take her maggot infested foot locker away. Far away.

The confused resident may babble, carry a doll or

teddy bear around with them, or even appear completely lucid. He or she may pace endlessly which we used to consider the early symptom of Alzheimer's disease. Sometimes the personality changes and memory becomes as a bubbling stew. Then again, the resident may have excellent short-term memory but no long-term memory. Again, it could very easily be just the opposite. If the resident is mildly confused, we prescribe activities that hopefully will help with the confusion. With marked confusion, a resident may pick out a bed partner and crawl into bed with him or her. This is quite a rude awakening for the resident in his own bed. In any event, we keep a very close eye out for the confused residents wherever they might be. They love to leave the facility. The resident might decide it is time for a cold beer and off to the store, he goes. It is an all-out emergency when a resident is missing. One case was a gentleman who was a severe alcoholic and very confused. He got out and he was found two or three days later dead, behind a Dumpster about two miles away, with several large empty bottles of rubbing alcohol strewn about him. We were not charged with his death by the state this time. The Alzheimer's unit was always locked but the front door of the facility was unlocked on the inside (by law). Some of the residents on the Alzheimer's unit are very crafty and will walk out with a doctor or clergy man who doesn't know the resident cannot leave the unit. Even the windows could have been a method of escape.

I got a call at home one night at about 7:30. This time two of our residents had left the center. We knew they were "sweet" on one another and we knew they drank. Everyone that could be spared joined in the search and finally, an aide who had been checking out the sleazy motel row in town found out from a manager of one the worst motels that our residents had just checked in. The director of nursing and I knocked on the motel room door and demanded to be let in. There they were: the female in bed and the male up, pouring himself a drink. We got them back to the facility but I had inner feelings about this that I didn't voice. I hated "rounding them up" like criminals when all they wanted was a little privacy away from the center. Residents are perfectly free to go out on pass, a legitimate pass with their families if they sign out and state when they will be back. Sadly, this was not the case with our love-birds as they both were residents on the locked Alzheimer unit. It was later found that they got out of the locked door with a family member who had been visiting another resident.

Chapter Seven

Meet the Department Heads

ADMINISTRATOR

The administrator gets in around 8 a.m. and works until about 5 p.m. Most have college degrees and they have successfully passed the state and federal Board exams to become licensed. Many are (or were) registered nurses. They are required to have continuing education hours in order to renew their licenses each renewal period. The number of these hours and the required subject matter varies from state to state.

The administrator should be out on the floor making rounds at least once or twice a day overseeing the staff and residents. He or she has many corporate policies to abide by (as well as hundreds of laws, rules, and regulations from the government) and if the corporation is large, the administrator will report to a regional manager (this position has different titles, depending on the corporation) who visits the facility regularly. The regional manager may have 10-13 facilities that he or she is responsible for and will visit more often if the administrator isn't adhering to the budget that is set in stone. They will also visit more frequently for other reasons that includes low census to budget census numbers, a bad annual or complaint survey by the state, a pending law suit; many reasons and most of them are definitely not good! When the regional just shows up on a routine visit, he makes rounds and looks at everything, even down to the bottoms of the pans hanging in the kitchen and the temperature log of the walk-in refrigerator. Actually, the administrator generally believes that what the regional is really doing is just wasting everyone's time but a report to the corporate office will be generated from his visit and he will have to have something to report, good or bad. Of course, I'm being facetious. Having been a regional myself, maybe I can get away with it. If that administrator is doing a good job, getting good surveys from the state and his census and bottom line numbers are up to corporate expectations, all is good. Add the pressure of having to be at top level functioning at all times to the everyday staff problems, possible family complaints, the usual problems with lost clothing, inability to hire good people; the list goes on and on and it's a wonder all administrators are not divorced. Many are. The administrator has to balance all aspects of the nursing home business with his/her personal life and let me tell you, it is not easy. When I was an administrator and I finally got home at night, I locked my door and felt that I was free, but at any time the telephone could end that feeling with one ring. Thankfully, that didn't happen too often.

But when the administrator is at home resting for the same big push the next day, he or she has no idea of what is going on in the facility. When I first started out as an administrator, I worried so much that I got up in the middle of the night to go to the facility and check what was happening. Sometimes all was good which left me tired the next day, but one time I fired the entire 11-7 shift for sleeping, which left me alone to care for 120 residents at 4 a.m. I don't have to tell you that shortly thereafter, many staff phones rang and I was more than tired the next day.

DIRECTOR OF NURSING

This head nurse usually works from 8 until 5 but the hours may vary depending on the need to visit the 3-11 and 11-7 shifts. This position reports to the administrator, is always an RN in a skilled facility and deals with all facets of the nursing department from staffing, adhering to all policies, the care plan system, training, ordering of nursing supplies and keeping within budget for same but most of all, quality resident care. This person has a very large job and it would take up two or three pages to list everything he or she does. The position carries a lot of authority but as is evident, a great deal of responsibility. There are tricks to the trade though such as proper delegation and constant follow up. There is no way that the director could possibly accomplish all the responsibilities alone. This position will have the inservice (education) and the care-plan coordinators report to him/her (generally RN positions) as well as all the unit managers (if there are unit managers included in the nursing staff). Occasionally, charge nurses will report to the director of nursing but more generally, they report to the unit managers. He or she should frequently hold nursing staff meetings that may address problems or explain new policies. It was always my rule that every member of the nursing staff must attend these meetings unless they were hospitalized. Sounds pretty tough but if you didn't come down hard on the staff you could be talking to four bare walls during your staff meetings. I must admit there were times when people were excused but they had to have a good, sound reason.

You may see the director of nursing and the administrator making what we called "clipboard rounds". They both carry a pen and paper on clipboards and they enter each room and look at everything, not only from a nursing standpoint but also from the housekeeping department and the maintenance department points of view. When the rounds are completed, the needs or repairs noted (it takes three or four hours), the findings are Xeroxed for the departments and highlighted with different colors for the different departments to take care of. They have twenty-four hours to make the corrections and report back to the administrator in writing that all has been taken care of. If the administrator and director of nursing are smart, they will go out and look at several of the findings to be certain they are all corrected.

You may find the director of nursing dressed in "scrubs" or in street clothes with a white lab coat on. It is a sure thing that you won't find her in starched whites with her school nursing cap perched atop her head.

SOCIAL WORKER

The social worker reports to the administrator and you may see this person doubling as the admissions coordinator. I hope you don't see that because both are more than full-time jobs. The social worker helps the residents apply for Medicaid, if needed and keeps track of the process all the way to approval. In an average center with a high Medicaid population, he/she will be working with the Medicaid office to approve ten or more residents for Medicaid. There is a log that must be kept describing where the resident is in the various phases of approval. It is not an easy job. He or she will also assist with insurance questions or problems, will become involved in the living will process if needed and in general will help all residents with social concerns and problems. In some centers, he or she will make appointments with outside physicians such as ophthalmologists and dentists and arrange for transportation. We always tried to keep these appointments down to a bare minimum if a family member cannot accompany the resident and certified nursing assistant must go with the resident. This has been discussed on previous pages.

It is impossible to name all the functions of a good social worker. Their tasks are varied but so important.

DIETARY MANAGER

This person is called a Certified Dietary Manager which means they have gone to school to learn the "ins and outs" of the proper handling of food and the correct management of a medical commercial kitchen.

It's not all about food but most of the residents think it is. The dietary manager generally is bound by a corporate contract to purchase food from a certain company, a big company. The bigger that company is, the more mistakes they make. All food deliveries have to be carefully checked for accuracy and the dented cans have to be separated and stored to be returned for credit. Sometimes the cuts and quality of meats don't arrive as ordered but cannot be returned because it must be used within the next two or three days. This one problem can lead to grumbling among the residents. Complaints from time to time are expected by the dietary manager even though the cooks do their level best to make the food look good and taste good, too.

No matter how experienced the cooks are, the food will still be labeled as "institutional". One of the reasons might be because the elderly have lost many of their taste buds and nothing tastes like it used to. Some residents complain about the food, tell their family members and then I have the family at my door. Some residents have poorly fitting dentures or no teeth at all. This always presents a problem because nobody likes pureed food, especially spaghetti and green beans.

Another reason could be that the menus are made by registered dietitians who are always mostly interested in nutrition and presentation. In centers that belong to large companies, menus are written at the home office and sent down for use. It can save the facility consultant registered dietitian and dietary manager a great deal of work not having to write menus but the problem is the menus might have been written by corporate dietitians in Chicago, Illinois for southern folk in Alabama or Georgia. All the menus have to be reviewed and frequent changes made and signed off by the facility's Registered Dietitian consultant. If you don't see a favorite on the posted menus, you can always request that it be added. Every part of the country has their cultural likes and dislikes so the menus must be altered. Then, of course, the food cannot be highly spiced as some residents prefer. Only a dietitian would serve green beans with spaghetti but those green beans always seem to be there. What's the matter with pizza, hamburgers with fries and spaghetti without the green beans every now and then? Of course, the residents do get hamburgers from time to time but it's just not the same as what you would get at home (unless the maintenance man had time to fire up the outdoor grill). Again, talking about spaghetti, why not a green salad, spaghetti, and garlic bread? I always ate the nursing home food and, naturally, some centers are better than others but I made certain that the dietary manager and I discussed poorly accepted meals and that the necessary changes were made.

The dietary manager coordinates staff parties, resident parties, and family council dinners in addition to their normal duties. And somehow they get it all done. The dietary staff makes sure there is a snack and fruit cart that tours the center supplied with cookies, puddings, juices, graham crackers and fruit. If your center doesn't have a cart, suggest it. The dietary staff prepares all the finger foods that are required by the

Alzheimer unit and keep the nursing stations supplied with food such as peanut butter, crackers, or soup for those residents who become hungry during the night. The dietary department also sends out an assortment of sandwiches, pudding, fruit, cheese with crackers, and cookies that is passed to all at bed time. It's amazing what they can do, and on a tight budget too!

The regulations for this department are very stringent, as they should be. Everything in the refrigerators has to be covered, labeled, and dated. Defrosting meat must take place in the refrigerator and it cannot be on a shelf over any food items. There are many logs that must be kept. It seems that every piece of equipment has a log attached.

When the state surveyors arrive, there is likely to be a registered dietitian with the team that will look at everything in the kitchen and comb the residents' charts looking for deficiencies. Each surveyor has an area that will be concentrated upon. There are registered nurses that review the nursing department. Add social services and maintenance and we have a lot of company during the annual survey. I have had only two or three facility-wide deficiency free surveys in my time but during one survey, I picked up a deficiency because the kitchen was too small. The surveyor that cited this deficiency was a good friend of mine, and the old building had been surveyed at least 28 times before through the years. I sputtered when I asked her why she had cited me on the kitchen. She just calmly looked at me and said, "I've never been in the kitchen before. You need more storage space." The registered dietitian was not along on this survey and it fell to my RN friend to survey the dietary department. We fixed this by adding several shelves since we couldn't add on to the building.

You will see dietary managers in every care plan meeting (in every facility) as they constantly deal with weight problems. (You really wouldn't think there would be weight losses with all the food the department puts out but there are and they are generally due to illness.) Frequently, the attending physician will order dietary supplements such as Ensure which is all well and good for a short period of time. Pretty soon, the resident won't touch the food and will only take the Ensure. It is sweet and tastes like a milkshake and requires no chewing. I am not a big fan of these supplements. They are expensive and I never thought they did much good. I liked to see the dietary director concoct high-calorie foods that would be accepted by the residents along with a good vitamin.

It is ever so important that every person at a table be served at the same time. There is no excuse in my book that allows a resident or two to sit and watch their friends eating when they are still waiting for their tray.

The dietary department frequently caters to special wishes of a resident. It may be goat's milk or it might be a certain brand of cereal, a particular type of juice generally not on hand or even a flavor of ice cream. I have seen a dietary department prepare a resident's favorite recipe for the whole house to enjoy.

When you tour the nursing home, notice if the residents have been taken to wash their hands prior to eating and notice how the meals are served. Restaurant style with the aides serving? Buffet? Family style? I have had the most success with Restaurant style where the resident's aide goes to the buffet line in the dining room, tells the cooks what is wanted and then the tray is promptly delivered back to the resident. The food was prepared in the kitchen then transferred to a hot/cold buffet in the dining room where the dietary personnel served the trays for the waiting aides. Not every center has this system. Every effort is made to give the resident what he likes but keep in mind that good nutrition must prevail so the resident cannot have tomato soup and grilled cheese sandwiches for every meal.

The dietary department can be good or it can be bad. If the latter is the case, the administrator should act promptly to replace the dietary service manager with someone else who is more caring for the residents as well as more professional. It's inexcusable for the food not to be the best possible. I once had a resident who said to me, "My next meal is all I have to look forward to." Sad, but frequently true.

I have spent a lot of time with this department because its quality is so vital for the residents' feeling of a certain level of contentment and satisfaction in their environment.

BUSINESS OFFICE MANAGER

This person is an extremely important member of the management team and can be found in the administrative part of the facility always surrounded by computer printouts and paper. (I might add that this position can have a big hand in the success or the failure of the administrator). This person generates statements for charges on the computer whether she sends them out or the home office does. Generally, the statement amount is due to be paid by the 10th of each month but most certainly before the next statement is issued. Inputting all the charges is a daunting job. She also bills all the government programs such as Medicaid and Medicare. One of her most difficult jobs, in my opinion, is dealing with insurance companies that never want to pay. This part of the job takes a great deal of time as insurance companies will do almost anything to keep from paying and some companies are worse than others.

Accounts receivable is a huge part of this job as well as dealing with a report called an "aging". This breaks down all resident accounts by amounts owed and will list amounts to be paid by Medicare, private, Medicaid, hospice and insurance. It will also indicate how far past due they are. The insurance companies because of their slow payment really hurt the aging and this report is reviewed and judged by all levels in the nursing home company from the business office manager all the way up to the president. The report is like a barometer indicating how good the administrator and business office manager are at doing their jobs.

Another problem she faces is the Medicaid-pending resident accounts (those who have not yet been approved for payment by Medicaid). In Florida, it has taken two to three months or longer to be approved by Medicaid even if the family is very prompt with all Medicaid's requests. If the family is not prompt and drags its feet, it may take three to five months. I've frequently seen Medicaid cancel an application for lack of family cooperation. In Florida, the Social Security income that the resident receives pays to the nursing home as the responsible party portion with exception of an amount usually less than $50 which is for the resident's personal use. This isn't very much particularly if the resident smokes. If the Social Security check comes to the family or the resident, sometimes it is spent and the nursing home doesn't get paid. This is a major problem. The Social Security check can be made to come directly to the center and this makes it easier on everyone. The amount for the resident is deposited to the resident's trust fund.

It is imperative that all families know exactly how Medicaid operates in their state. You probably have guessed that the business office manager and the administrator spend a considerable amount of time collecting past-due accounts. In my centers, I always collected the past-due private accounts and the business office manager did the insurance and other types of accounts such as Hospice.

The business office manager can also be in charge of the front office personnel that perform such jobs as accounts payable, secretarial work, managing trust fund accounts for the residents, reception work, workers' comp, and benefits for the employees, running police background checks on potential employees, etc. There is one hell of a lot of work that goes on in the "front office".

ACTIVITY DIRECTOR

This important person is responsible for so many things. Let's say he or she has 120 residents with diverse interests or in many cases, no interests left at all. Throw in an Alzheimer's unit to service and this person has a tremendous job to do every day. I always cringed when a non-knowing person would call the activity director the "play lady". When most people think of what nursing home residents do for fun, Bingo comes immediately to mind. This is partly true; they love their Bingo but there is so much more. There is entertainment from the community that the director brings in and there are generally a lot of children that come to sing, especially at Christmas time. So many, in fact, that I always enjoyed playing "Scrooge". The reason behind this was not because I dislike children but rather because they brought in their winter viruses and drippy noses. Every time they came we had a little rash of respiratory illness.

The activity director prepares a giant activity calendar decorated with the theme of the month or season that is prominently displayed for all to see. There should be at least 6 - 8 activities scheduled per day for the general house. They may include a reminiscence group, a sing-along, exercise, group trivia, arts and crafts, current events, the always-loved Bingo, movies with popcorn (or other treats) and other activities that the residents have requested. If the facility is fortunate to have an assistant activity director, this person generally works on the weekends keeping the activity program moving right long seven days a week. Weekends are always lonely for the residents. If the facility doesn't have this position, sometimes an aide will put on two or three activities a day. In any case, there are always puzzles, magazines, and movies for the residents' use.

For the bed-bound residents, the activity director makes up baskets of interest for that particular resident to keep in their room

The Alzheimer's activities are different. They may consist of listening to music, watching TV or even having their hair brushed and nails done. The attention spans are so short and it is very difficult to engage them in a regular activity. Frequent fun-foods are provided, and are always enjoyed the most.

MAINTENANCE

This position is usually held by a man but I've heard of lady maintenance personnel in nursing homes. His job is what might be labeled as "humongous". He takes care of the air-conditioning, changes filters and light bulbs. He does the fire drills and writes up the minutes, takes care of the emergency generator, and tests it frequently. He purchases maintenance supplies and equipment, and is held to a budget. He paints, he repairs, and daily he checks the temperature of hot water coming out of the taps in residents' bathrooms and makes sure that the water is hot enough in the kitchen. He logs almost everything he does. He is extremely good at unclogging toilets (every maintenance man cannot understand why nursing staff members are unable to unclog a toilet) and he also does a lot of preventative maintenance. At least he is supposed to. A good place to find him is up on a ladder replacing ceiling tile or up on the roof replacing what ever they replace on the roof. I've often thought the roof was a good place to take a break. He generally carries a beeper with him as he seems to be everyplace all the time. (There is one thing a maintenance person really hates and that is if a department head buys a new desk, bookcase, or whatever for their office. He feels that everything has to come to a halt to put the thing together and we generally leave him alone in times like these.)

ADMISSIONS COORDINATOR

As most nursing facilities belong to large corporations, the push is always there to fill the house to capacity. The pressure is very intense at times for the admissions coordinator and the administrator. The person must be an expert on Medicare, Medicaid, and all forms of payment including insurance so as to be able to help the families at the time of admission. Frequently, the admissions coordinator will take baskets of goodies or even lunch to hospital discharge planners in hopes they will steer some potential residents their way. Visits are made to the assisted living facilities hoping for referrals and also visits to physician offices are made again in hopes of direct referrals to the particular facility. The admissions coordinator makes many telephone calls and is one of the busiest people in the center knowing they can be replaced by someone more productive and with more contacts. This person along with the family does all the admission paperwork and an admission can easily last an hour or more.

HOUSEKEEPING & LAUNDRY

And last but certainly not least, there is the director of housekeeping and laundry. This position is much more complex than the average person would imagine. There are many infection control and other nursing policies that must be followed to the letter. This director must make constant rounds checking behind her housekeepers and looking for "high dust", dust behind doors, proper cleansing of bathrooms; this list is unending. The director must also follow up on the floor personnel to be sure all floors are clean and shining, but not slippery. Schedules are made and posted but if there is a call-in, the director generally has to take over that job for the day, and maybe longer. The laundry will run at least fifteen hours a day with two shifts and the amount of laundry they put out is staggering. Not only must they wash the soiled bedding, they have items from nearly every department that must be washed and dried. Now, add most of the residents' clothing and instantly, these hard-working laundry personnel have gained a lot of respect along with the housekeepers whose job is never done.

These are the top department heads and they are not listed by importance to the team. Every one of them is vital to the optimal level of service in the nursing home. When a new resident is admitted, each department head should stop by and introduce themselves, and tell the resident and the family members how they can be reached. There should be a bulletin board by each resident's bed and it should contain the activity calendar, the latest newsletter, a regular calendar and extension telephone numbers for named department heads. I posted my home number on every room bulletin board but not once did I ever receive a call.

Chapter Eight

The Alzheimer's Unit

The reason for an Alzheimer's unit is to separate the victims of this terribly regrettable disease from the general population of the facility so to allow them the specialized care they require. This unit is generally locked because of the Alzheimer residents' penchant for pacing and wandering. It truly is amazing how these unfortunate residents can find a way out. Over a very tall fence, climbing a tree, walking out of the unit with a visitor who doesn't suspect a thing. Most of these residents that are so active generally are in the earlier stages. Sometimes they look like you or me, but most are always ready to either pace or leave. Later on, it's a different story. They die. I believe that many victims are misdiagnosed as they do not all follow the same path through the illness. There really only is one positive way to diagnose Alzheimer's and that is on autopsy of the brain.

I'll not forget my first experience with Alzheimer's disease. I received a patient in one of my centers in southwest Georgia via ambulance from Atlanta with the diagnosis of Alzheimer's disease. The year was 1978 or 1979. My director of nursing burst into my office and said, "We just got a patient in with Alzheimer's disease. What the hell is that?" I had absolutely no clue but I called our medical director, Dr. Christmas. He had no idea either. He said for me to "cool it" and he'd make a few calls. Within the hour, he was back to me and said, "It's just a fancy name for OBS (organic brain syndrome)." I don't think anyone really knew what OBS meant but it was a dandy "catchall". During this resident's stay with us, we watched this very handsome man with beautiful blue eyes deteriorate right before our eyes. He had been a trial attorney in Atlanta but he couldn't keep the job in his firm. He drifted with odd jobs to Florida where he became so disoriented that he was picked up on the street and confined to a psychiatric hospital. They somehow found out that he was from Atlanta and he was transferred there to another psychiatric hospital that did their best to find his wife. She had gone undercover, but at least they were able to make a diagnosis of Alzheimer's disease. The gentleman gazed with his clear, aquamarine eyes at his caregivers and at me on my visits to his room. For a very short time, I thought I saw a glimmer of intelligence deep in the eyes that followed me. Soon, though, the eyes were completely blank. He would no longer squeeze my hand. Then one morning, I saw on the 11-7 shift report that my first Alzheimer victim had departed this world. We all missed him and we in-serviced (trained) the nursing staff about Alzheimer's disease that we would see much of in the future. We couldn't guess at the coming onslaught of Alzheimer patients.

I opened my first locked Alzheimer's unit in Florida and never had a deficiency from the state through four or five annual surveys, except for one. The aides didn't follow the activity calendar that was posted in the unit's common room. I might add here that a video was playing but the calendar said it was "Sing-Along-Time". Nobody bothered to ask if the residents had not responding to the Sing-Along, which they did not, so the aides turned on the video. This was no doubt what happened after our investigation of the deficiency. The state didn't care and would not remove the deficiency.

I was so fortunate to have a nurse unit manager named Donna for the Alzheimer's unit. She became quite well-known for her talents and traveled the state to help other centers start their units. Donna kept the unit housekeepers in line and her unit was the cleanest in the facility. She devised activities with the activity director for her 30 residents and upon observation, one could observe an occasional gleam of remembrance or interest in the usual blank eyes. This unit's residents received special finger foods and lots of high calorie and protein foods as the Alzheimer victim has special caloric needs. There was always a lot of peanut butter, puddings, and fruit available. If the resident could not feed himself, he would be fed carefully to be sure there was no weight loss or choking. Hydration was watched so carefully and juices plus special drinks came from the kitchen on regular intervals. Water was constantly encouraged and the intake of liquids (as well as food) was monitored and charted.

The unit was very special. The nurses, the aides and the great unit manager did a fantastic job. The residents, so confused, so 'out of everything' were gently and lovingly cared for. The staff members in the unit were all best friends and totally dedicated to their charges. They had parties for the residents who didn't recognize a party but they greatly enjoyed the special party foods and ice cream. They always wanted more.

Was there a downside? No, there wasn't, but this does not mean that all Alzheimer's units are of this quality. When touring this unit, you should see clean residents in clean clothing. And you must be sure that you look at the fingernails and hair. You may see people in a state that you've never seen before. There will be no restraints but please don't let this type of resident frighten you so that you won't notice the fine points of excellent patient care. Look at what everyone is doing. Are the residents comfortable? I had one resident in the unit that had a pet dog who was always at his master's feet whether in the bed or on the floor. We took care of the veterinary bills for the elderly dog and he was one of our star residents except he didn't have Alzheimer's disease. The resident was allowed to take his dog outside on potty runs but he always came back with his beloved dog. I believe this friendly resident somehow realized he was fortunate to be able to keep his dog with him. I firmly believe that both would have soon died if separated.

Talk to the staff and the unit manager to see what ideas they may have for your Alzheimer's victim. Ask questions. Look at the quality of housekeeping. Do the floors shine? Are they clean? Notice the interaction between the staff and residents. If you decide to place your loved one on this unit, please be a frequent visitor on all three shifts. Get to know all the staff and maybe even bring some cookies or treats from time to time. They'll love you. The nursing staff is always starving.

Chapter Nine

Ins and Outs of the Nursing Department

STAFF MEMBERS AND STAFF NUMBERS

Even though I have loved them all, I sometimes wanted to wring their necks. Take the nursing aides for example. We never let the staffing numbers fall below what the state required but sometimes we had a couple of extra aides working. Every time we were down to the required numbers, the aides would whine to the family members or to the residents, "We're working short". The family members, who had no reason to disbelieve the aides, would become nervous and even angry. Then they were at my door demanding why the aides had to work short and was their mother receiving the proper care? At nursing staff meetings, I went over the required staffing ad nauseum but to no avail. I spoke to the families during their meetings. All this to no avail. If an aide said, "We're working short", it was gospel and there was nothing the director of nursing or I could say to convince them that the nursing staff was not running short.

Let me show you how to figure nursing staffing. I could never teach the certified nursing assistants, but then they didn't want to learn either. It was easier for them to whine about working "short". The following will pertain to a skilled long-term care facility (SNF). There are different levels of nursing facilities depending on what level care they provide. The skilled center is what we are dealing with here. There are three levels of nursing staff employees: RN (registered nurse), LPN (licensed practical nurse), and the C.N.A. (certified nursing assistant). Each level has a number of hours per a 24-hour period that must be worked. Let's ASSUME the average national number of residents in a skilled nursing facility is 95.6. This is one of the numbers we will be working with. In your state, the staffing time required may be different from what I'm quoting here (national averages). The formula is the same though. Let's do a little arithmetic. It isn't hard. Remember, we're using national averages.

RN's: 30 minutes per resident x 95.6 residents = 2868 minutes or 47.8 hours per day. We divide this by an 8 hour shift that the RN works and we find that 6 RN's must be on duty in a 24-hour period. Not too hard, huh?

LPN's: 48 minutes per resident x 95.6 residents = 4589 minutes or 76.48 hours per day. We divide this by the 8 hour shift they work and we find that 10 LPNs are needed on duty in a 24-hour period.

C.N.A.'s: 138 minutes for each resident x 95.6 residents = 13193 minutes or 220 hours per day. Many centers have 7.5 hour shifts for the C.N.A.s, but some have 8 hour shifts. We will use the 7.5 hour shift here and divide the 220 hours x a 7.5 hour shift and we come up with 29 C.N.As needed for the 24-hour day. The heaviest staffing is on the day shift and it tapers down to the night shift. The arithmetic is easy. Find out your state's staffing requirements and then on any given day, IF YOU KNOW WHAT THE CENSUS IS, you will be able to tell if the nursing staff is staffed to meet the requirements.

You will need to ask the director of nursing what her staffing pattern is for each type of nursing personnel. If there are several admissions one day, the staffing requirement might rise a bit. If there are several discharges on a particular day, the staffing requirement may be a bit lower. This is figured on a daily basis and staffing is generally adjusted to what is required by law. I know that you won't be bamboozled by an aide that complains, "We're working short!!" There are, of course, centers that staff higher than required. I never had this luxury myself.

Occasionally, even though all employees are required to have rigorous police background checks, a thief will be hired. This person likes expensive perfume, money left on the bedside table, and Christmas or birthday presents. It is quite difficult to catch them as they are very crafty. One time, before the background checks were required, I went so far as to put a lady cop undercover as an aide (with instructions to not do anything aide-wise) on the 3-11 shift, where I was having so much trouble. The cop put a $50 bill halfway down a container of cotton balls in a resident's room and then she watched. At the end of the shift, the thief had not been apprehended but the $50 was gone.

Every now and then, even though they know it is against policy, a staff member will ask a resident for money. They are taught almost continuously that they may not accept gifts from residents or family members, nor can they ask a resident for anything. This act goes against all regulations and policies by which the nursing home operates. It calls for immediate termination of the staff member. If a family member wishes to bring cookies or candy in, it must be for the nursing shift, not one individual.

Speaking of termination, one of my best aides working on the 11-7 shift had a resident that screamed the entire night. The aide must have snapped mentally as she stuck a rolled up sock in the resident's mouth to stop the screaming. Immediate termination.

Sometimes, the aides must endure what no human should have to endure. They are spat on, cursed at and some even worse things can and do happen to them. I don't know how they do it, but at least 98% of them do, and remain loving and caring at the same time. Working in a nursing home gets into your blood and if you asked, most of the staff would tell you that they wouldn't do anything else.

I had one sad situation that also called for immediate termination. We noticed food items, cans of Ensure, and the like missing but we just couldn't catch the thief. My son volunteered to get on the roof and watch as the workers left the building after the 3-11 shift. I was parked in the parking lot, also watching. We caught an excellent aide who had placed a bag of food items taken from a resident's room into a bush outside the side door to be retrieved at shift change. When she got her bag, we had her. She became very emotional and told us that her husband was a drunk and taking food from the nursing home was the only way she could feed her children. I felt bad and I believed her, but a facility cannot feed the world.

Licensed nurses are cats of a different color. None of them learn any management skills in their training and then are expected to manage the work and behavior of six or eight aides. Mostly, they are excellent and pick up the people management skills quickly but then there are always some that think that their only real duty and purpose in life is to pass meds and chart. Passing of meds always comes first.

I hope that I have not been too hard on the nursing staff. The above described problems are few and far between. In my last center, there were aides that had worked there for 27 years and they were wonderful. I made very good friends with many of the nurses and aides through the years. They all work hard and don't make much money. But they care.

One time, I had an RN that I will call Mary Ann. She had been an officer in the military. She was so experienced and so intelligent but we found that she was on drugs and alcohol. She had such severe problems. Her father had just died an early death and her husband had developed a severe disease. She never had any money because of her husband's super-expensive drugs. One day, the director of nursing invited me into her office and asked me to close the door; always a good sign of trouble in the air. She told me that the narcotic counts at the back nurses' station were not correct and hadn't been in a while and then, as if that were not enough, she told me that she had strong evidence that Mary Ann was the one taking the residents' narcotics. After listening to the evidence, there was nothing to do but call Mary Ann in and confront her with it. She was full of denials, and appeared hurt that she was suspected. We told her that we were taking her to a lab for a drug screen. She didn't like it but had no choice. I took her in my car but first, before we left the building, she said she needed to go to the bathroom. I said, "No, come with me. We're leaving right now." The nursing director had called the lab and told them we were on our way. Once there, she was handed a specimen cup and sent to the bathroom to obtain a urine sample. Three times, she brought out a specimen. Three times, the lab tech refused it because it was the wrong temperature. (Urine is body temperature. Mary Ann's was far too cool.) I finally said in my sternest of voices, "Mary Ann, stop with the games. Take this cup and do it right this time. This is your last chance." She meekly accepted the fourth cup from the tech. This time the tech accepted her specimen. She knew she'd been "busted". She stayed at home for a couple of days until I received the lab test results. Almost everything imaginable was found. I wondered how she could even function well enough to walk. I called her into my office and the director of nursing and I discussed the findings with her. She was so embarrassed and afraid for her nursing license. She definitely had a right to be fearful. She swore she would enter the Impaired Nurse Program for addicted nurses as we required. Not only that; she swore to enter Alcoholics Anonymous. She immediately entered both groups and we had the proof of it. Now it was time, actually past time, to let my company know what had occurred. The president came on the line and said, "Well, I hope you fired her." I answered, "No, she was ill and is now receiving treatment. Her drug room and medicine cart keys have been taken and I feel this is the best thing to do for her." The president was not happy and said, "I hope you know what you are doing!" I nodded, hoping so too, and hung up.

Mary Ann was the model nurse following her 'fall from grace'. She was a fine, well-educated nurse and she fully recognized where she had gone wrong. After many months, because her performance was so good (and after the Impaired Nurse Program "said so"), her keys were returned and later she was promoted to assistant director of nursing. She functioned surprisingly well in this role and did much to better the staff. In the meantime, I had been having rather severe problems with the director of nursing. Finally, I had no choice but to terminate her employment. She was devastated but business has to be business and she was doing a piss-poor job. She excelled at the financial end of her job dealing with invoices, ordering and keeping within her budget. Certainly, all these things were necessary but as the overseer of fine patient care, she lacked significantly and didn't know what the hell her staff might be doing, as she so seldom made rounds. The staff lost respect for her and even started laughing at her behind her back. She was not doing skin checks for decubitus ulcers (bedsores) to verify the reports that she was given by the charge nurses. And the number of sores began to climb at an alarming rate.

Here I was without a director of nursing. Since I was an RN and had been a director of nursing, I could hold it together for a while, but my job as administrator was very demanding and by law, I couldn't function in both positions. I called Mary Ann into my office and asked her to consider the job. She thought about it, talked to her husband and said, "I can't do it. I'm afraid that I won't be a good director because of my past and besides that, I don't know how to be a director." I promised her that I would teach her a few little tricks of the trade such as "Delegation and Follow-up". She reluctantly accepted the job, and became the finest director of nursing I ever had and she even amazed our company. She decided that she might like to be an administrator a year or so later and since I was a "preceptor" for the State of Florida (trained by the state to train new administrators), I trained her along with the very fine social worker of the center for a year and they passed their state and national board exams with flying colors. She didn't stop there. She became a consultant for a major long-term care company and even went so far as to be promoted to Regional Manager with many facilities in her charge (even though she had never been an acting administrator) and now she is being considered for a vice presidency. Shortly after she finished her training, I began a year's training for her husband. Now, they both are in the business, he as a fine administrator and she as a Regional Manager. They both pull down the big bucks and live in a country mansion with their golden retriever. This is the greatest success story of my career. I learned many important lessons from Mary Ann and I'll never get over being so very proud of her.

I have many stories about nursing home nurses going the extra mile. How the long-term care nurses differ from hospital nurses is that they generally have time to know and love their residents. Hospital nurses turn the beds over to new patients all the time. While they may be kind (or maybe not), they just don't seem to have the compassion of the long-term care nurses. Hospitals are not nearly as regulated as nursing homes. This can be noticed by used syringes left at bedsides, trays of food left too far away for the patient to reach. I'm not knocking hospital nurses by any means, but the geriatric long-term care nurses are as highly trained in their field as most of the hospital nurses. Long-term care nurses are trained to act more independently. They talk to physicians most every day but only see each of them monthly on a usual basis when they visit their residents. Mostly, the medical director checks in weekly. They are also frequently far better in patient care since they know their residents so well.

The medical director, who is always an MD, is a paid consultant. The duties are varied and include signing off on all new policies, monitoring patient care rendered by both physicians and nurses, attending meetings where the MD expertise is required and assisting with the general health of the staff members.

The medical director will see the new admissions that may be assigned to him as well.

The regulations that dictate to long-term care are voluminous and every agency seems to have their own set. The feds have theirs, sometimes the state has theirs, the nursing home companies have their stringent policies and the nursing home itself has still more. Let's not forget the Ombudsman Committee who works for the resident in solving problems. If a resident has a problem with anything in the facility, there are posters in the center with the telephone number of the local Ombudsman Committee for the residents or family members to call and make their complaints. This will cause a member of the committee to visit and look into the complaint. If the complaint is serious enough and is found to be valid, the Ombudsman will call the state surveying agency to come in and deal with the problem. I was usually able to convince the residents to come and tell me their problem and I took care of it to their satisfaction. But there are always residents who do not wish to speak to anyone in the facility.

It's a tough life for an administrator, demanding perfection from the center and knowing there is no such thing as perfection in a world full of people. We strain, we stress, we plan, and we analyze results every day. Are we successful? Sometimes. Sometimes not, but mostly, I think we are. Nursing homes vary in quality and always will. Why? One big reason is lack of experience in management. The poorer facilities also figure the state surveyors won't find their problems if they try desperately to get things straight and running smoothly right before the unannounced survey. This is not the way to do it. You must be survey-ready every day of the year or you might need to find another business. Yes, it's most difficult to maintain that high level of quality every day. Yes, sometimes a facility will slip because a system breaks down but it can be fixed. It is much easier to run a center this way than trying to guess when the surveyors will arrive at your front door. What do they do if the survey is early? Oh me, there might be many, many deficiencies. I have heard of survey deficiency reports being more than eighty pages long. Definitely bad news for all concerned.

Chapter Ten

Family Members ~ God Love 'Em

There are several different types of family members:

"I'M THE ONE HERE THAT KNOWS IT ALL"

This poor soul haunts the halls looking for problems waiting to become major disasters. She strongly feels that all medical care involving her loved one, and perhaps other residents as well, should be checked through her. She faithfully attends all of the care plan meetings where she and other family members are allotted a private quarter hour to assist in planning the care for the loved ones. All department heads that have anything to do with the resident's care and social life are there and the person in charge is almost always an RN. As each family member arrives at the meeting, they are told that there are only fifteen minutes to get a whole lot done, so if they wish to make complaints or comments, would they please wait until the meeting is over and then those involved in the area of the problem would be more than glad to talk to them. This particular family member heeds none of this and proceeds to take an hour or more with her laundry list of complaints and well thought-out plans for improving the services of the facility. The RN in charge can appear to be rude while trying to stay on schedule, but it does no good. Those families who were patiently waiting for their scheduled time were long gone and feeling put out by the care plan committee especially since most of them had jobs to return to.

She memorizes the attending physician's visit schedules and she's always there waiting for him with her trusty drug dictionary in hand (no doubt she also has several geriatric medical textbooks on her bedside table at home). The physician does what he can to avoid her but it just doesn't work. If the physician elects to change a med, change the dosage, add a med, or even change the rate of the tube feeding for her resident, she demands to know exactly why, which is her right. She goes too far though when she checks new meds in her drug book while standing in front of the doctor. He just walks away with a curt, "Good Day". Sometimes she follows him to another resident's room still questioning, and talking a mile-a-minute.

This is one of the types that threaten to "call the state" if she thinks something is "going on" or that something is awry. She can and she does. Then, here come the state surveyors who fine-comb her complaint and other matters that may be discovered during their visit. They may stay only a day but it isn't infrequent for them to scrutinize the facility for three days. It is no fun and it is a period of extreme high stress. In my experience, those complaint surveys were mostly deficiency free but if a facility is not tending to business, woe be unto that nursing home.

How does the staff feel about this family member? They're scared and sometimes so afraid of repercussions that the resident may not receive the planned care. This can present a major problem and even though the management and charge nurses watch out for this to happen, it is impossible to watch every C.N.A. every minute of their shift. I've had suspicious family members hide a tape recorder in a room hoping to catch the aides in some non-professional activity. I've even had family members watch through the window at night. It is quite understandable that the aides feel very paranoid and subconsciously tend to stay away from the problem. One may think, (and I'm quite certain the family member feels this way) that a highly visual, threatening family member will cause the staff to do a better job. No so. Definitely not so. A no-win situation.

"WHAT CAN I DO TO HELP?"

This family member is a joy. She comes to share meals with her loved one and visit with the staff up and down the halls. She knows them all by name and gives compliments when they are due. If she experiences a problem or has a request regarding her resident's care, she approaches the charge nurse in a friendly manner and discusses the matter with intelligence. If the charge nurse does not handle the problem to her satisfaction, she makes an appointment with the administrator and director of nursing. Many administrators, me included, do not require an appointment and are available at any time for family members. I included my home telephone number in the admission packet and asked either the resident or family members to call me at any time, day or night.

She will frequently bring in home made brownies or cookies for the staff members, who are always ravenous. Nursing facilities often raise money for various charities and this type family member is always right in the middle of the events such as yard sales or bake sales, and working hard. Sometimes she has problems with the facility but she doesn't scream at the staff and berate them publicly.

This person helps with resident birthday parties and special events often suggesting innovative ideas such as a live tree-planting ceremony complete with an engraved plaque as a memorial to a resident who has passed on. Her help, given with a positive attitude, can only make the nursing home a far better place for all to live. She trusts the facility and she realizes all of the staff members are human and things can go wrong, but she also knows those in charge will take care of the problem immediately and to the complainant's satisfaction. This is not to say that this person will condone any problems with care that she sees. We would not want this and always welcomed another pair of eyes to see a problem as we never could be in all places at all times. A word from her was all that was needed to start the ball rolling.

The center loves this family member and her loved one. The staff will bend over backward doing extras for this person who treats them with dignity, respect and recognizes their hard work.

"I KNOW WHAT YOU'RE DOING AND I'M GOING TO GET YOU!"

This family member is so difficult because there's no way to break down her barrier. She will hide tape recorders in her mother's room and will bring movie cameras into the center even though she knows they are prohibited because of loss of privacy for any resident caught on the tape or in a picture. A resident must sign a release if he or she might be photographed.

If a resident is unable to sign, that resident may not be photographed. We have to be very careful with this as nursing homes take many pictures of their residents and often make collages to hang in the dining area or in the activity room.

This family member generally is looking for a law suit and doesn't mind telling this to the staff members. A weight loss on a resident will send the family member to an attorney even though the problem is documented, care planned and approaches to the problem by nursing as well as dietary are carried out. There are many attorneys out there who make lots of bucks on nursing home cases. They advertise their services in all media sources to make the "cruel nursing homes pay for what they did to the frail and elderly resident". Thanks to the legal climate, it is horribly difficult to defend a nursing home, even though it may be a clear cut and dried situation where the nursing facility was definitely not at fault. Suits were settled out of court because the attorneys for the nursing home didn't want the facility to face the jurors. Why? Nursing homes have all the positive publicity of a leprosy outbreak. Ask anyone on the street, and everyone has a horror story about a nursing home. And shame on the nursing home if this family member's loved one falls. Though not a usual practice, I've seen family members sue and leave their loved ones in the facility. This is always a sure tip-off that the family is only looking for money. I've even had a nursing assistant staff member sue for the care that her grandmother received. This staff member worked the hall where her grandmother lived. She didn't remove her grandmother either.

"I'M SO UPSET. I DON'T SEE HOW I CAN LIVE. MOMMA ALWAYS TOLD ME SHE WOULDN'T GO TO A NURSING HOME."

This family member is guilt-ridden for untold reasons. I always had a box of tissues on my desk. I have had a woman faint in my office during her mother's admission. (Another reason why I think RN's make the best administrators). This family member would weep buckets at her mother's bedside. This was doing absolutely no good for her mother, and perhaps even instilling fear. If her mother were up to being assertive, she might have said, "Quit with the hysterics. I'm here. Let's just see if I can get better so I can go home to my cats." This doesn't happen very often though as the mother may well suffer from timidity as well. I frequently counseled family members and reminded them over and over again that they had to take care of themselves first. If they did not put themselves first, they would be no good for their loved ones. I dealt with family member guilt every day for twenty seven years.

AND THEN ~ THERE'S ME

Yes, even though I was the administrator, the boss and the 'captain of the ship', my mother developed a raging case of ovarian cancer and couldn't live alone any longer. She became one of my residents. I don't know if she listened to me over the years (she always laughingly called nursing home residents "victims") but she was the perfect resident. The nursing staff absolutely adored her. Not because her daughter was the administrator but because she was so considerate and thankful to the staff. Frequently, staff members would take their breaks visiting with her in her room. She never complained and her only real request was to have a cinnamon roll every morning for breakfast. When the nursing home staff finds a resident who cares about them, they will do anything for that resident.

My father and his wife were somewhat of a different story. My parents divorced when I was seventeen because he had begun an illicit romance with his current wife, Peg. Daddy and Peg had gone downhill extremely fast mainly because of his increasing blindness, her alcoholism and refusal to care or cook for him. They, too, could no longer live in their home. They came to be admitted in my facility but not without arguing. Their real problem was that they were both alcoholics, but I got an order from their doctor for two drinks in the evening, which I fixed for them. I hid the bottle, but Peg always found it and became very drunk. This put a tremendous strain on the 3-11 shift but they put up with her because of me, I guess. They shouldn't have had to put up with this and I tried different hiding places, but she still found the bottle. Finally, I left the bottle in the locked med room and that was the end of that. Soon, my Daddy died in July and my Momma followed in October. Peg was with us for about a year after that but every month marked a downhill trend to where she was comatose at the end.

My mother loved one of our nursing home pets, "Fifi", a male guinea pig (he always thought of himself as a lady guinea pig) that lived in a glass aquarium tank. When Momma's death was imminent, I moved "Fifi", cage and all to her bedside, but Momma was just too far gone to even look at "Fifi". The last word I heard from Momma was when I asked her how she felt. She said, "Peachy". That was my mother. She never gave up but the cancer took her the next morning. I analyzed my staff and my mother's care and determined without a doubt that her care was the same as the other residents received. The best. I was so proud of my staff.

"BIG BIZ BINDLESTIFF"

These are the family members, usually men but

sometimes women, who will come to admit their mother or father and lay down the rules. "Call me for this. Don't call me for that." It is explained that we have regulations that dictate when we will call and if a nurse feels it necessary, she will call. This family member backs down but makes it clear that it will be impossible to visit very often. We always gave that resident extra attention because sure enough, the family member hardly ever showed.

However, there's still another type and when I close this manuscript, I'll no doubt think of more family member types but I think you get the picture. The following is the worst that I've ever encountered.

"THE ABANDONER"

I've had so many daughters and sons who have left their responsibilities with me. Sometimes I had a suspicion but it didn't deter me from taking an admission that needed to be placed.

The awesome responsibility of a very ill loved one added with the guilt of admitting the resident can cause a family member to run without a forwarding address. It never took us long to find out that the resident had been abandoned and it hurt so bad when the resident asked had we heard from the son or daughter. I became incensed with this problem and did my best to track the family members. I only found one and when I started in on her, she told me she was close to death herself from breast cancer. She didn't want her mom to know. There was nothing to say, I began visiting her mother every day and doing what I could do to make up for her daughter. A stand-in is never the real thing though.

This case was an exception. Mostly, it was getting the resident on Medicaid, having the Social Security go to the nursing home as required and then poof. "Bye Bye". "I'm outta here!" Too bad. Oh, so too bad. No matter the guilt, there is never a reason to abandon a human being, even to a loving facility.

Chapter Eleven

Resident Rights

I have taken these resident rights from the internet and will comment in italics on some of them as we go along. A copy of these rights will be given to every new admission. If you do not receive them, please ask for it.

"The Nursing Home Reform Amendments of OBRA 1987 require that nursing facilities 'promote and protect the rights of each resident.' The resident rights must be displayed in the nursing home along with a contact number for the state's Long Term Care Ombudsman (a third-party resident advocate)."

The general goals of the law are:

QUALITY OF LIFE

The law requires nursing homes to "care for the residents in such a manner and in such an environment as will promote maintenance or enhancement of the quality of life of each resident." A new emphasis is placed on dignity, choice and self determination for nursing home residents;

Our "social model" nursing home helps provide this.

PROVISION OF SERVICES AND ACTIVITIES

The law requires each nursing home to "provide services and activities to attain or maintain the highest practicable physical, mental, and psychosocial well-being of each resident in accordance with a written plan of care which is initially prepared, with participation to the extent practicable of the resident or the resident's legal representative."

It is hoped that family members will attend each care plan conference. You should be notified when a conference is scheduled so that you may make arrangements to be there. The center should make every effort to have the resident at his/her care plan conference but if this is not possible, such as the resident being bed-bound, the resident must have the care plan explained. In my experience, this is best handled by the Social Worker taking the care plan to the bedside, explaining it and answering any questions that the resident may have. If possible, we have the resident sign the care plan stating that it has been explained.

When family members attend the care plan conferences, it should always be remembered that several residents will be discussed in the time allotted for the meeting. There may be other family members waiting for their time to enter the care plan room. Each resident receives about fifteen minutes and all time must be devoted to creating or upgrading the resident's care plan. If there are patient care problems and/or complaints, these are best handled by appointment with the appropriate department head, the administrator or the director of nursing. It could easily be that an appointment would not be necessary. All you have to do is ask. These professionals want to hear of your concerns and problems. If they are not aware of a problem, there is nothing they can do about it.

PARTICIPATION IN FACILITY ADMINISTRATION

The law makes "resident and advocate participation" a criteria for assessing a facility's compliance with administration requirements.

The best way to achieve this is to have a very active Resident Council that meets regularly. This council may invite the administrator or any other department head to attend and answer questions. Concerns and complaints are aired and sometimes even a few compliments are handed out by the council. All residents may attend and are encouraged to attend this meeting. Resident officers are elected at convenient times and staff may only attend if invited by the council. Minutes are always taken stating possible problems, and copies are given to the appropriate department heads who, in turn, will answer in writing to the council what the plan is to take care of any problems that have been voiced. Family councils can take place in the same way.

ASSURING ACCESS TO THE OMBUDSMAN PROGRAM

The law grants immediate access by ombudsmen to residents and reasonable access, in accordance with state law by ombudsmen to records; requires facilities to inform residents how to contact ombudsmen to voice complaints or in the event of a transfer or discharge from the facility; requires state agencies to share inspection results with ombudsmen.

As stated, the Ombudsman Program is a "third-party resident advocate." You will see posters showing the telephone numbers for the ombudsmen prominently displayed in the center. The Ombudsman Committee stands ready to assist any resident that may need intercession for whatever reason. Always, I have found them to be positive and very helpful. They also conduct an annual survey of their own.

SPECIFIC RESIDENT RIGHTS

Rights to Self-Determination: Nursing home residents have the right:

* To choose their personal physician.

* To full information, in advance, and participation in planning and making any changes in their care and treatment.

* To reside and receive services with reasonable accommodation by the facility of individual needs and preferences.

* To voice grievances about care or treatment they do or do not receive without discrimination or reprisal, and to receive a prompt response from the facility.

With regard to the right "to choose their personal physician", not all physicians visit nursing facilities and you would need to inquire from your personal physician if he will follow the resident at the nursing home and abide by the laws pertaining to physicians visiting nursing home residents. This includes visiting generally at least once a month. There are usually two or three physicians that practice in the facility, one being the medical director, as a general rule. If your physician says that he cannot follow the resident, you certainly can choose one of the physicians that do practice in the facility.

* To organize and participate in resident groups (and their families have the right to organize into family groups) in the facility.

Personal and Privacy Rights: Nursing home residents have the right:

* To participate in social, religious and community activities as they choose.

* To privacy in medical treatment, accommodations, personal visits, written and telephone conversations and meetings of resident and family groups.

* To confidentiality of personal and clinical records.

Rights Regarding Abuse and Restraints: Nursing home residents have the right:

* To be free from physical or mental abuse, corporal punishment, involuntary seclusion or disciplinary use of restraints.

* To be free of restraints used for the convenience of the staff rather than the well-being of the residents.

* To have restraints used only under written physician's orders to treat a resident's medical symptoms and ensure his/her safety and the safety of others.

* To be given psychopharmacologic medication only as ordered by a physician as part of a written plan of care for a specific medical symptom, with review for appropriateness by an independent, external expert.

Restraints including bed side rails are not used in most facilities in Florida, because of the terrible accidents associated with residents attempting to crawl through them. As a Florida State surveyor once told me, "Residents have the right to fall and break a hip." Can you believe it? True enough! I strongly advise questioning the use of restraints in the facility you are considering. Keep in mind that some medications may be regarded as restraints. This is one reason why the purpose of the medication is always noted on the medication sheets in the charts.

Rights to Information: Nursing homes must:

* Upon request, provide residents with the latest inspection results and any plan of correction submitted by the facility.

You should see inspection (survey) results prominently posted in the center along with the written corrections. These results are public record and can even be found easily on the internet (Medicare.org), however if a resident wishes a copy, it should be given at once.

* Notify residents in advance of any plans to change their rooms or roommate.

In a facility with Medicare certified beds, there is always a problem keeping those beds available for a Medicare admission. Only a certain number of beds are certified and they must be contiguous (there are centers that have all their beds certified). If a Medicare bed is certified, any pay type can occupy that bed but a Medicare resident can ONLY be placed in a Medicare bed. For those centers that are very interested in a high Medicare census, they may try to move your Medicaid or private pay resident out of a Medicare bed. Your resident or you do not have to agree with this and it is your resident's right to remain where he/she wants. If the resident wants to move, then that's great for everyone.

* Inform residents of their rights upon admission and provide a written copy of their rights, including their rights regarding personal funds and their right to file a complaint with the state survey agency.

* Inform residents in writing, at admission and throughout their stay, of the services available under the basic rate and of any extra services, including, for Medicaid residents, a list of services covered by

Medicaid and those for which there is an extra charge.

* Prominently display and provide oral and written information for residents about how to apply for and use Medicaid benefits and how to receive a refund for previous private payments that Medicaid will pay retroactively.

You will want to ask for a list of services and charges such as for the beauty shop.

With regard to the above as it states "refund for previous private payments that Medicaid will pay retroactively", this is a bit confusing. When Medicaid is applied for, there are many things that have to be furnished to the Medicaid office such as bank statements. Sometimes, family members do not get the job done quickly enough and a long period of time will elapse between the admission date and the time the resident is approved for Medicaid. During this time the resident might be on private pay status with the family paying the monthly rate for the care. At the time of approval, Medicaid will go back and pay for those months and the family will receive a refund from the facility. As you can see, it certainly behooves you to be very prompt with Medicaid's requests as the private rate is not cheap. There are, of course, those facilities that will wait until Medicaid pays from the time of admission. It's extremely important to ask this question prior to admission if your loved one will be on Medicaid.

Rights to Visits: The nursing home must:

* Permit immediate visits by a resident's personal physician and by representatives from the licensing agency and the Ombudsman Program.

* Permit immediate visits by a resident's relatives, with the resident's consent.

* Permit visits "subject to reasonable restriction" for others who visit with the resident's consent.

* Permit ombudsmen to review resident's clinical records if a resident grants permission.

Transfer and Discharge Rights: Nursing homes must permit each resident to remain in the facility and must not transfer or discharge the resident unless:

* The transfer or discharge is necessary to meet the resident's welfare and the resident's welfare cannot be met by the facility.

* Appropriate because the resident's health has improved such that the resident no longer needs nursing home care.

* The health and safety of other residents is endangered.

* The resident has failed, after reasonable notice, to pay an allowable facility charge for an item or service provided upon the resident's request.

* The facility ceases to operate.

Notice must be given to residents and their representatives before transfer:

* Timing: At least 30 days in advance, or as soon as possible if more immediate changes in health require more immediate transfer.

* Content: Reasons for transfer, the resident's right to appeal the transfer, and the name, address and phone number of the Ombudsman Program and protection and advocacy programs for mentally ill and developmentally disabled.

* Returning to the Facility: The right to request that a resident's bed be held during hospitalization, including information about how many days Medicaid will pay for the bed to be held, the facility's bed-hold policies and the right to return to the next available bed if Medicaid bed-holding coverage lapses.

This is something to keep in mind. If a Medicaid resident goes to the hospital and remains a long period of time, chances are the Medicaid bed-holding will have expired. Make a note to inquire at the business office how many days Medicaid allows in your state. I have seen a resident transferred out of the hospital to another center because no beds were available at his home center. Of course, they are entitled to the first open bed but it probably won't be the one occupied before hospitalization.

Orientation: A facility must prepare and orient residents to ensure a safe and orderly transfer or discharge from the facility.

Protection of Personal Funds: A nursing home must:

* Not require residents to deposit their personal funds with the facility.

* If the facility accepts written responsibility for the resident's funds, it must:

a. Keep funds over $50 in an interest bearing account, separate from the facility account. Amounts may vary by state.

b. Keep other funds available in a separate account or petty cash fund.

c. Keep a complete and separate accounting of each resident's funds, with a written record of all transactions, available for review by residents and their representatives.

d. Notify Medicaid residents when their account balance comes within $200 of the Medicaid limit and the effect of this on their eligibility. Again, check you state's requirement.

e. Upon a resident's death, turn funds over to the resident's trustee.

f. Purchase a surety bond to secure residents' funds in its keeping.

g. Do not charge a resident for any item or service covered by Medicaid, specifically including routine personal hygiene items and services.

If your resident is covered by Medicaid and he/she is approaching the amount of the Medicaid limit, it would be an excellent time to shop for needed items for the resident such as clothing or even a new TV. All receipts must be brought to the person in the front office handling the trust accounts. Remember, this money belongs to the resident and I have had several misunderstandings with families that spent the money on personal items for themselves.

We most highly suggest that residents not keep cash in their rooms. If they want a Coke or a haircut, the money can be obtained from the person handling the trust funds for the facility.

I also want to point out that allowing jewelry to be worn by your resident is asking for big trouble. The worn wedding ring can slip off a finger and end up in the laundry, never to be found. If your resident wants to keep jewelry at the center, it can be locked up in the office safe. There is always a log of everything contained in the safe.

Protection against Medicaid Discrimination. Nursing homes must:

* Establish and maintain identical policies and practices regarding transfer, discharge and the provision of services required under Medicaid for all individuals regardless of source of payment.

* Not require residents to waive their rights to Medicaid and must provide information about how to apply for Medicaid.

* Not require a third party to guarantee payment as a condition of admission or continued stay.

* Not charge, solicit, accept or receive gifts, money, donations or other consideration as a precondition for admission or for continued stay for persons

eligible for Medicaid.

I have never seen discrimination toward a Medicaid resident. The nurses could care less what pay source the residents have and if you were to ask one of them what pay source your resident was, he or she would have to go to the chart and look at the face sheet. Face sheets are not things that nurse look at unless they need to find a telephone number to contact a family member, etc. (Naturally, they know if a resident is covered by Medicare as the resident would be in a Medicare certified bed and there are certain other rules that apply to the Medicare resident that they are aware of.) There is nobody in the facility that cares. Some would say that the administrator should care as the center isn't receiving what a private pay resident would pay but let's face it, there aren't that many private pays out there and Medicaid is now paying a fairly respectable rate. A lot of centers have census problems and are happy as clams to get a Medicaid admission.

There are a few other things that are required that aren't mentioned above and they are:

1. *You have the right to purchase drugs from your pharmacy of choice. However, the medications must be delivered very timely to the center and packaged according to the medication system that the center is using. You may inquire as to the system during admission and then check with your pharmacy. Usually they cannot package the medications for the particular system. Medications must also be able to be delivered on a "stat" basis which means right away, day*

or night and on holidays.

2. You have the right to send and to receive mail unopened.

3. You may share a room with a spouse, if medically feasible.

4. You may have a secured space, with a key, for safekeeping of small personal items. All centers do not automatically offer this but it should not be a problem for them to accommodate you.

Chapter Twelve

Medicare and Medicaid

It is important particularly with Medicaid that you check with your state and the admissions coordinator as to what the rules are. Most of the numbers, etc. I have given are from Florida and I have used them only as examples.

I have described what payment sources you must have in order to be admitted to a skilled nursing facility. But let's do it again:

1. You may be covered with Medicare - see below

2. You may be covered for Medicaid - see below

3. You may pay privately.

4. If the facility is VA certified, certain veterans may

be referred to the facility by the VA.

5. Long-term care insurance. Please see the note at end of the chapter. I've tried to be very succinct with these subjects. Both Medicare and Medicaid-programs are very complex and have lengthy manuals describing what they cover and what they do not cover. If you have further questions about Medicare, you may go online at: http:/www.medicare.gov/longtermcare and hopefully, you can find what you are searching for there. Incidentally, you may find all the nursing facilities in your area with the number of survey deficiencies and more information that will make your decision so much easier when trying to find the right facility. This information should never take the place of the facility tour though and you should tour several before making your decision. The social worker, administrator, or business office manager can also help by furnishing you the information you need. Don't ever be afraid to ask if you don't understand something.

MEDICARE

Most folks don't know the difference between Medicaid and Medicare. Medicare Part A is what you will come to the skilled nursing center with if you need skilled care, and if you qualify. It is federally funded.

Medicaid, on the other hand, is a program for people with limited income and resources. It is a joint federal and state funded program. We generally tend to think of Medicare as federal and Medicaid as state. A person covered with Medicaid can also enter the skilled nursing center. That's okay if you don't know the difference between the two. I didn't either until I got in the business. Those covered under Medicare will have a red, white and blue card from the government that you will have to show to everyone that admits you to a hospital or to a skilled nursing center and even the girl behind the desk when you see a new physician from the day you receive the card, and forever more. There is Part A and Part B. Part A doesn't cost anything but Part B does. We will limit our discussion of Medicare to Part A. When all program requirements are met, Medicare Part A helps pay for:

* Care in a hospital

* Care in a skilled nursing center following a hospital stay

* Home health care

* Hospice Care

Let's talk about coverage:

To be covered under Medicare (and by the way, it is the skilled nursing facility that decides if coverage may be provided using Medicare's very stringent guidelines), the following conditions must be met.

1. You require daily skilled nursing or rehabilitation services that can only be provided in a skilled nursing facility. (Example: If you can get physical therapy next door to where you live and you can get there, it would not be covered in the nursing facility). Also note that you must require DAILY skilled nursing care or rehab services.

2. You must have been in a hospital for three days in a row (72 hours) not counting the day of discharge before admission to a skilled facility.

3. The reason for which you are receiving skilled nursing care or daily rehab must be the reason why you were in the hospital or it could be from a problem that arose in the hospital.

4. You must be admitted to the skilled center within thirty days after leaving the hospital.

5. A medical professional (MD) must certify that daily skilled nursing or rehabilitation is necessary.

Now, let's talk about benefit periods:

Coverage for care in hospitals and skilled nursing facilities is measured in "benefit periods." In each benefit period the number of days Medicare will help pay for inpatient hospital or skilled nursing facility care are limited. Once this limit has been reached and you are still residing in the center, you will have to pay the private pay rate for each additional day of care as Medicare will no longer pay.

A benefit period of 100 days begins the day you are admitted to a hospital and it ends when you have been out of a hospital or skilled nursing center, and not having received skilled care for 60 straight days (including the day of discharge). A note here: Consider the fact that you might have received skilled care while at home. Remember, you must have the 60 days free of skilled care. Once you have exhausted one benefit period, a new benefit period can begin. There is no limit to the number of benefit periods you may have. Remember, a new benefit period for the skilled center always begins with the 3 day hospital stay.

Part A pays the full cost of covered services for the first 20 days. All covered services for the next 80 days are paid by Medicare except for a daily coinsurance amount.

It may be that you won't be covered for the entire 100 days. As an example, let's say the resident is receiving daily skilled rehabilitation services. The rehab department has reached their goals and cannot help the resident any further. They will then discharge the resident from their service. So frequently, facilities that have little experience with Medicare will send you a "cut letter" telling you that the resident is no longer covered by Medicare. Where they might have failed is by not looking at the skilled nursing that the resident might be receiving. He might be tube fed, which is always skilled. He might be receiving wound care for a bedsore (decubitus ulcer) which is also skilled. If there are absolutely no skilled services received, Medicare will no longer pay. Skilled services must be provided by a licensed nurse or professional therapist. There is such a thing as coverage for the aggregate of the unskilled services which requires a licensed nurse to manage a lengthy care plan for a resident who is receiving care by C.N.A.s. I, personally, have never used this to cover a resident but I have provided coverage when the licensed staff was training a diabetic to give his own insulin injections and for that matter any other service that the resident will provide for himself at home.

What happens if you are discharged from a skilled nursing facility and later must be readmitted? If you come back within 30 days, Medicare will resume paying for your care until you have used up your 100 days. The care must be for a condition treated during your first stay. Remember again, that if you are not receiving skilled services by a licensed nurse or professional licensed therapist, Medicare will not pay.

Not all nursing homes are skilled nursing facilities. Many other homes offer custodial care such as help with bathing, toileting, taking medications, eating, etc. Medicare never pays for custodial care.

When you receive services by Part A Medicare, you do not have to file a claim for payment. The hospital, skilled nursing facility, or other provider from whom you received the services will file the claim for you.

What happens if you disagree with the decisions concerning your Medicare benefits? There is an appeal process that will be sent with the letter from the facility stating the resident no longer is covered. It is a straight-forward form but if you should require assistance with it, the social worker or business office manager can help you fill it out and send it in.

This has been brief mainly because you will receive a great deal of information about Medicare when you place your loved one, and there is always the internet.

MEDICAID

This description will necessarily be brief because Medicaid programs vary from state to state. The resident's income limits for Medicaid also vary.

Please call your State Medical Assistance (Medicaid) office to see if you qualify. For more information about Medicaid, you may call 1-800-MEDICARE (1-800-633-4227) to get the telephone number for your State Medical Assistance Office.

If your loved one is paying privately in a skilled center, their money won't last forever and it would behoove you to make an appointment with the local Medicaid office to talk to them about applying before the funds are depleted.

LONG-TERM-CARE INSURANCE

I don't think I need to explain that long-term care insurance must be purchased before the condition appears that takes the person to a nursing home.

Just a note as there are so many varied policies, and you would need to talk to a representative that deals in this type of insurance. Make sure the agent is licensed in your state. You can also find "A shoppers Guide to Long-Term Care Insurance" by calling 1-800-MEDICARE to get the telephone number for your State Insurance Department.

If you can find a reputable long term care insurance company, I personally would highly recommend that you think about purchasing a good policy. I have seen families wiped out financially when there was no other option than to pay private rates.

Chapter Thirteen

A Word About Money

People complain at length about the price of nursing home care. And yes, as I said, I've seen long-term care costs eat up a lifetime of savings in spending down to be eligible for Medicaid to pay the nursing home bills. Private daily rates may run between $175.00 and $300.00 or more per day depending on the part of the country you hail from. Besides this, we have medications, physician visit fees and possible therapy charges. If the resident has Medicare, it can be billed for certain items but even if you only had to pay the daily room rate, it's still a lot. The percentage of private residents in a facility is usually small compared to the Medicare and Medicaid residents and we can certainly see why, but there are times when there is no other choice. Again, may I recommend that you look into purchasing a GOOD long-term care policy, before it is needed. There are those who have different ailments, for example, who require oxygen only at night (myself included) that cannot be insured.

Now, let's look at this in another light.

What does the resident get for this daily rate?

He/She receives a bed in a semi-private or private room. The private room is the most expensive. There are some older centers where you will find "ward rooms" with three or four beds but these are falling by the wayside.

Nursing care is high on the list. A very personalized nursing care plan is designed on admission that considers current problems and even potential problems such as guarding against weight loss, decubitus ulcers (bed sores) beginning or healing those that exist from a hospital stay. The initial plan is developed with the family members' assistance and updated on a regular schedule or when there is a change in the health status of the resident, or a hospitalization. The nurses and certified nursing assistants are trained in geriatric nursing and they receive in-house education called inservices on a set schedule. It would be impossible to list all the duties of the nursing staff but they are many and they are varied - from cleaning up an incontinent resident, to feeding a resident that cannot feed himself, to guarding against falls and many other things.

He/She receives three nutritious meals a day, all snacks, and even food during the night if the resident is hungry. The dietary department keeps lists of each resident's food likes and dislikes and they, hopefully, go beyond the call of duty to honor these wishes. There is always a cup of coffee available and the dietary staff frequently goes out on the floor to talk to residents about how the food is being accepted.

Your resident will have a full activity schedule tailored again to likes, dislikes and even to abilities.

Social Service helps with bank account problems, Medicaid, insurance policies, and even personal problems. They go out of their way to ease a resident's worries. I once had a male social worker that I saw coming toward me in the hall. He was only in stocking-feet. I said, "Bill, where in the world are your shoes?" He smiled and said, "Mr. Spence didn't have any shoes so I gave him mine." He was the best social worker I ever had but he had a "problem". He was too handsome and most of the female staff was in love with him. One even went so far as to stalk him when he was off duty.

We must not forget our Housekeeping staff and the laundry staff. The housekeepers keep the floors clean and gleaming, the rooms dusted and the bathrooms sparkling. The laundry staff will do your personal laundry, and launder all the bedding, towels, and dietary linen. You would not believe the amount of clean linen they put out every day.

And then there is the maintenance man who keeps everything humming along smoothly (except when he decides it's time for a fire drill. It is NEVER at a convenient time). Most maintenance personnel are very happy to make minor repairs for residents. I had one a long time ago that just loved to fix broken jewelry; inexpensive costume jewelry.

We cannot leave out Administration. Among many other things, the administrative staff manages patient trust funds for the residents. A family member may leave money for their loved one to have their hair done or the resident may receive monthly checks from different sources. These funds are managed from the front office with statements sent out regularly to the residents and family members. The Business Office Manager is always there to explain whatever it is that you might not understand.

In a 120-bed facility, there will be approximately 100-105 employees, most dedicated to doing the best job possible for the residents. Salaries are the highest expenditure that a nursing home faces.

And then there are utilities (big bucks), the lawn care

company, the plumber who had to come and retrieve a towel from a toilet, the mortgage payment, taxes, insurance and it goes on and on.

The general consensus of opinion is that nursing homes make big money. That is absolutely not true. The costs to run a facility are astronomical. Toward the end of the year, the administrator and the company put together a budget that will run through the next year. It is made up of historical costs for the previous months of the current year. We add small percentages to utility figures as they seem to always go up and we have to increase on the salary line because raises have to be given. Another thing is that if the competing facilities have raised their level of pay, every facility probably ought to do the same or some of the staff will just leave to work for the highest paying facility. The overall costs, hopefully, will be fairly constant from the previous year with added percentages where needed. The biggest thing that will affect the budget bottom line is lower than budgeted census numbers. When the census dips, the administrator starts to sweat and look for ways to cut back a bit. We don't want to do that and sometimes we can't.

We call it a "pennies business" because all of our costs are measured in "per patient day" numbers. Department heads such as the dietary service manager, the director of nursing; anyone that spends money for supplies had better know what their costs are running

per patient day. Years ago, a lot of years ago, I could
feed a resident for $1.56 per day including three good
meals a day, snacks and treats. I've no idea what it's
running now but it has to be a lot more. Keep in mind
that big ticket items such as food, cleaning chemicals,
laundry soaps, etc. is bought on negotiated contract
prices from the various vendors.

Department heads use what we call "spend down
sheets" whereby the amount that is budgeted, let's say,
for nursing supplies is entered on top of the sheet.
Every purchase is subtracted from that budgeted
figure and department heads learn fast how to make it
through the month on what money they have to spend.

Chapter Fourteen

Abuse

It's time we talked about abuse. What exactly is abuse? My dictionary defines it as:

To use wrongly or improperly.
To treat in a harmful, injurious. or offensive way.
To speak insultingly, harshly, and unjustly to or about.
Commit sexual assault upon.

There are more definitions, but we get the picture.

Where do we find abuse? It's in the workplace, in the home, in the church, on the roadways, in prisons, hospitals, nursing homes, child care centers, and we find raging animal abuse in all walks of life. Who commits these atrocities? As much as I hate to say it, we all have been guilty of abuse in our lives. In the human race, children, the elderly and infirm are recipients to the worst degree. How can this be? Is it because some undiscovered wrinkle in our brain knows that certain people cannot defend themselves because of childhood, age, or disease? Do we subconsciously feel that the aged and ill have lived their lives and should step aside so that we may live ours and not to have to concern ourselves or care about the non-productive ones in our midst? Are we really only animals that will cull our ranks to be rid of noncontributing members? No, we don't want to think this is possible. And we don't want to think of ourselves as mean-spirited for even thinking such a thing. Maybe it's only because we are human and our tolerance and patience wears thin with the constant care and giving to non-providing members of the human race.

Let's get a bit more specific. When opening a new facility, I had to go in on a Mother's Day because of several call-ins by nursing assistants. It is good for an RN administrator to work as an aide every now and then so as to not forget the terribly difficult work that the aides do day in and day out. It was lunch time and the trays for the bed bound and those who required feeding had arrived on the floor. We passed those trays belonging to bed-bound residents and got them ready to eat. I then went to get my first tray that belonged to a woman who had not fed herself in months and was steadily losing weight. I began feeding her and she would have none of it. No matter what I did, she just turned her head. I finally took her head and held it straight toward me attempting to get the spoon in between her tightly clenched teeth. I knew I had two more trays waiting to be fed to residents. By now the food would be cold and I'd have to reheat the trays. Something snapped in me and I had an exceptionally fervent desire to hit this lady in the face. How I overcame that desire and came to myself, I do not remember but I do know that I came within an instant of committing one of the worst kinds of abuse. Mental strength caused me to back away, but does everyone have this degree of mental strength? I've never forgotten it and I hope that I never will.

Let's say you are caring for your mother, your husband or maybe even your child who is desperately ill and perhaps even comatose. The physician does not predict any change for the better in the patient's condition. If you are a saint, you can give the finest care, devote your entire life year upon year to this person, forsaking friends, family, and all normal life activities. In the end, how would you be able to describe your health? That person that you have given your life to may even outlive you. This is so wrong. You must take care of Number One which is yourself or how are you going to be able to care for the loved one in even a limited way if you have lost your health? Caring for yourself means not giving up your entire life for another being. How many of us are saints? We snap because we are exhausted, we haven't been outside in a month, and we have not had any supportive family life. What could we do to keep this from happening? Not a damn thing. Most abuse occurs in the home with children and the elderly receiving the brunt of it. People can snap like dry twigs. They do it all the time.

My daughter, Liana, who worked for a publishing company, had to visit an author who was wheelchair bound from polio to discuss her book. During the conversation, the author told stories of verbal abuse from the her husband and caregiver. Liana was truly shocked and said, "That is just not acceptable" and went on to tell the lady that she didn't have to put up with that kind of treatment.

The lady nodded her head and then said, "No. No." She then looked into my daughter's eyes and said, "You have a lot to learn about life."

My daughter was truly distressed at this and came to me about it. I told her if she suspected abuse, she needed to report it to the abuse hotline. There is a law that requires reporting but she said to me, "I was only told about this. I didn't witness any abuse". Who knows? An investigation of this lady's potential abuse may have accelerated the level of abuse from her caregivers in payment for the embarrassment of an investigation. Therefore, if there is continuing abuse, will an investigation actually make it much worse? But since the lady stated she had been verbally abused, was my daughter wrong to not have reported it?

Hospital abuse hardly ever gets reported because most families and patients really don't know what constitutes abuse. We tend to look up to these nurses and doctors in white as almost superhuman. Believe me, they are not. They too, can be guilty of abuse. Frequently, they violate patient confidentiality and even cause patients more physical problems than they came into the hospital with. A supper tray that is set on an over-the-bed table that is too far for the patient to reach? The nurses not turning a bed patient every two hours? Physicians and nurses talking about a patient's medical problem within earshot of visitors and other patients? Used needles and syringes left on the over-the-bed tables without being properly disposed of in the red Sharps container?

Abuse happens everywhere but most of us try to do our level best to find solutions in every setting. I cannot say that I am aware of hospitals investigating subtle abuse cases probably because, as I have already said, it has not been reported. In the nursing home setting, families, residents, and even other staff members do not have any problem reporting what they think is wrong and there are many avenues for reporting. And I've always been glad of it. There was an occasion where I reported to the state what I considered abuse by one of my own C.N.A.'s. I dealt with her and so did the state. She ended up losing her

C.N.A. certification. All personnel must go through a thorough police background check that explores past arrests, convictions, etc. It is never good to hire until the background check is received. When this became law, it really helped us because we certainly didn't want to employ someone with a background of theft or domestic abuse.

Nursing homes usually have three shifts: 7 a.m. to 3 p.m., 3 p.m. to 11 p.m. and 11 p.m. to 7 a.m. Some facilities are a bit different but we'll use these times. If abuse is going to occur, it often happens during the dark hours. Not because the staff person knows he or she won't be seen but rather because this is the time that some residents, particularly the Alzheimer victims and the dementia patients, will try the patience of a saint. And yes, during the time of the full moon, it is worse. The following is an example: Each resident has a call bell that is clipped to their pillow so that the resident can easily summon the nurse if they require pain medication, have a need to go to the bathroom, etc. These call bells can ring every 30 seconds or more, often from the same resident. The aides and nurses are constantly checking and finding that there is nothing wrong and there are no evident needs. What this resident might be experiencing is loneliness but more probably confusion. The dead of night adds fuel to an all ready simmering level of confusion. The nurses and aides feel that they're spending their whole shift on this one resident with the call light. What does an enterprising young aide do to take care of the matter? She disconnects the call light. Oops!! ABUSE. What would happen if the resident really did experience an emergency episode and the call light was turned off? And I already told you about another aide, my best 11-7 aide, that took all she could from a lady that screamed through the entire night and then she snapped and shoved a dirty sock in the resident's mouth. ABUSE. Both of these aides were immediately terminated. How could the nurses and aides have handled these situations without resorting to abuse? Long before their nerves were completely frazzled, they could have gotten the resident up and into a robe for a ride in a wheelchair to the nurses station or dining room for a cup of hot chocolate or even a bit of conversation. Just being with people always seems to help the confused person. I have soaked their feet in warm water and that seemed to help considerably. Why do the nurses not do any of this? Some think they're too busy and many of them have succumbed to the old trap that claims so many long term care nurses. They begin to feel that their only job is to pass meds and chart. They leave all the good, old fashioned nursing care to the aides. I have had a licensed nurse tell me that she doesn't have time to supervise her aides because she has too much charting and other duties to attend to. On the 11-7 shift, most residents don't require anything except turning every two hours if they can't turn themselves to prevent pneumonia and bedsores. But the screamers and the ones who have found that their call lights will bring someone to the bedside can take the time of these aides for the whole shift while the nurse sits with her coffee, charting at the nursing station. I am being unduly harsh on the licensed nursing staff here and I know that. There are many, many fine nurses who truly care for their residents and would do anything for them and these nurses are the majority. But we sometimes are cursed with those who look upon the 11-7 shift as a highly paid babysitting job with aides to do the real work. We finally are able to weed them out but it's a never ending problem.

A good way that abuse can be decreased is by the aides, residents, nurses and family members all bonding as much as possible. Family members coming to visit and making friends with the staff goes a long way. If there are concerns about resident care, the administrator and director of nursing must stand ready to hear of your concerns and take care of them to your satisfaction. You should be able to visit each of them at your convenience, however, it is always better to make an appointment because there might be a meeting scheduled at the time you arrive or one of them may be out of the building.

I have heard of rape in the nursing home and I've heard of fire ants that killed a lady in her bed. I've heard of a snake in a resident's bed but these are stories that one hears and I've no idea if they are true or not, but I'm sure the lawyers were there on the spot. The hospitals also have their share of stories and it is one of the problems that have always plagued health care.

Abuse will be with us as long as this world continues to turn. We work to correct it all the time but it still happens occasionally. We are dealing with human beings.

Afterword

I thought I'd finished this book but then it occurred to me that if another administrator picked up this book, he or she might chuckle and say, "No nursing home can do all this!", and then go blithely back to their desk and continue to direct a so-so nursing home resulting in a lot of unhappiness and problems. I wish this administrator and those that fall into this category would take this book and use it as somewhat of a model to increase the quality of care in his or her facility. It is also my wish that administrators will not tell a prospective family member that what is written in this book is "pie in the sky" and cannot possibly be done. My biggest wish is that administrators that pick this book up are already doing a admirable job. **There are many fine homes out there with great administrators. All you have to do is find them.**

I must make sure you know that how I describe practices and policies on what should be done in nursing homes is how I did it in Florida and Georgia. I have no doubt that there are far better administrators than I was but I'm hopeful that the poorer functioning centers will get on the road to success and give the best care possible besides making their residents and family members happy and content.

You have to be careful when looking up centers with their State survey deficiencies on the internet. Some states are not as tough as others. I will repeat: This does not replace the personal tour and using what you've learned here to determine if a center is right for your loved one.

If your family member is already in a center and what you've learned here is not being done, I suggest that the Family Council speak with the administrator of the center about the things they'd like changed. If he/she makes no changes, find the next step whether it is a regional manager or the home office and take your suggested changes to them. I beg you to do this.

I wish I could say that my facilities were the very best. I can only hope that what I did made my residents and family members healthier, more content, confident and most of all, happier.

www.ingramcontent.com/pod-product-compliance
Lightning Source LLC
Chambersburg PA
CBHW051527170526
45165CB00002B/634

* 9 7 8 1 4 6 3 5 7 3 7 6 8 *